Financial Stability for the Disabled:

A Self-Help Guide for Social Workers, Caregivers, & Persons with Disabilities

By
Shelley Qian
Kayle Paustian
Austin Mardon

Edited by

Lawrence Dommer

A Golden Meteorite Press Book.

Published by Golden Meteorite Press.
126 Kingsway Garden
Post Office Box 34181,
Edmonton, Alberta, CANADA.
T5G 3G4

Telephone: 1-(780)-378-0063
Email: aamardon@yahoo.ca
Web site: www.austinmardon.org

Interior formatting & cover design by Alexa L. Guse, 2012

Library and Archives Canada Cataloguing in Publication
Financial stability for the disabled : a self-help guide for social workers, caregivers, and persons with disabilities / by Shelly Qian, Kayle Paustian & Austin Mardon ; edited by Lawrence Dommer.

ISBN 978-1-897472-41-5

1. People with disabilities--Canada--Finance, Personal.
2. People with disabilities--Services for--Canada--Finance.
I. Paustian, Kayle II. Mardon, Austin A. (Austin Albert) III. Title.

HV1559.C3Q25 2011   332.0240087'0971   C2011-905981-9

Financial Stability for the Disabled:

A Self-Help Guide for Social Workers, Caregivers, & Persons with Disabilities

By
Shelley Qian
Kayle Paustian
Austin Mardon

Edited by Lawrence Dommer

Edmonton, Alberta

Contents

Introduction

This book will be presented as a collection of short stories dealing with people with disabilities and the various services and benefits that may be available to the disabled. It is a self-help book that will contain the most common and accessible methods for managing finances for the disabled and those with low-income in a manner that is easy to read and understand. It is a compact manual that will give you an idea of where to begin when someone you know is or has become disabled. At the end of each chapter you will find a detailed description of all of the programs mentioned throughout the chapter as well as how to apply to the applicable federal programs. Because each province and territory has their own separate, distinct, and ever-changing programs for people with disabilities, it is impossible to cover all of them within one book alone. Therefore, we have specifically chosen four topics that deal with the life stages of a disabled individual and the federal programs available during these times. We have also chosen to include four provinces of interest to give you an idea of what types of provincial or territorial programs may be available.

addressing

the complications of

disabled

individuals

Chapter 1

Chapter 1
Addressing the Complications of Disabled Individuals

It is important to point out that everyone is "Temporarily Able-Bodied." This refers to the belief that a person is only able to perform daily tasks without physical or mental difficulty for a portion of their lifetime. This is not to say that a person will become defined as disabled, but merely, unable to perform the tasks to the extent that he or she was able to before. Usually, this condition does not improve or will not improve to the point where one can say they are back to 100% of their previous capacity. It is noteworthy to say that many people find that becoming disabled brings about greater difficulty than they initially believed possible. For many, the disability can become much like a second job, since you are required to attend various types of therapy, spend time with your doctor and other health care professionals, fill out forms, as well as discuss your illness and various medications that you may be required to take. The allocation of time for appointments and time for financial planning can lead to difficulties in finding a job that will suit your scheduling needs. This, in turn, leads to previously able-bodied individuals accepting jobs that are significantly below their previous pay grade, if they accept them at all.

Within our country, there are currently 3.6 million Canadians with some sort of disability. This number increases as the age of mortality increases and as the population increases as a whole. The Government of Canada does not have a set definition for what a disabled person can or cannot do, nor what their disability means to their life. It is for the disabled individual to figure out what he or she needs and how to achieve it. As such, it is not uncommon if at one point in our lives we find ourselves becoming more dependent on loved ones for assistance. Sometimes, the dependency is financial in nature. The problem of a financial hardship is that most individuals have a hard time being able to understand or find suitable resources to solve it. The majority of us will never think that this dilemma will ever chance on ourselves or our family. Others cannot afford to protect themselves from the financial hardships by applying for disability insurance. Because we cannot predict the future and we choose not to prepare, this book will attempt to address those that have been affected in the present to see if we can change the outcome of the future as well as broaden our knowledge to help others.

The goal is to ensure that our audience is aware of the various types of government funding available for disabled individuals. Although we cover a broad spectrum of funding and support programs, it is often not enough to allow one to meet acceptable living standards. Often, when someone becomes disabled they are forced to file for bankruptcy due to the costs associated with maintaining their previous lifestyle as well as the costs of supporting their disability. Unfortunately, not many people will realize this until it is too late. We have, therefore, also felt the need to address some additional lifestyle changes that may allow you to adapt to living on low income.

It is important to realize that there are many costs ranging from the financial to the emotional that can come with being disabled and this book has been designed to help you with each. We firmly believe that becoming disabled does not mean that your life is altered. You will be faced with making many sacrifices along the way but the tips included are intended to help you find a compromise, point you in the right direction, and hopefully, give you more time adjust to your disability.

We want this book to provide you with information to help you on your journey but by no means have we been able to unearth everything available for disabled Canadians. This book should be used as a guide to start you on the path of improving your life or the lives of others. It will no doubt open your eyes to many of the financial programs you may or may not have thought existed and we hope that the tips and tricks you have picked up throughout your read will enable you to become more independent and help you live a richer life. It is our intention to, not only provide you with information, but also hope and encouragement while we walk you through the struggles and trials of our character's as they deal with their disabilities.

When James was in the womb, we knew he would be a child with a physical disability that he must live with for the rest of his life. When the counselling had healed the heartache and taught us how to become mentally stronger, we began to prepare to deal with our son's disability. Even though he may not have the full use of his body, we were going to make sure he was loved and well-provided for so that he can learn to feel like a normal child, teenager, and adult. However, it was just as important that he learn valuable lessons and have the self-esteem, mentality, and confidence to be an important part of society and to maintain and provide for himself when we no longer can.

Being the grand-daughter of a late entrepreneur, I had been raised with stories around how my grandparents had struggled to make ends meet when raising my father, without forfeiting his education. One of the most important lessons my grandfather passed on to our family was not how to be rich, but to manage with what we have. "Give a man a fish and you feed him for a day. Teach a man to fish and you feed him for a lifetime." We had never been lucky enough to be given the fish, but we had been taught well.

The Government of Canada website is a basis point for new immigrants and current Canadian citizens searching for information or support on taxes, health care, disability, employment, and more.

having a child

child

with disabilities

Chapter 2

Chapter 2
Having a Child with Disabilities

We knew that having a child who was disabled would be very different than having one who was not, therefore it was imperative for us to start looking at ways to raise a disabled child and prepare ourselves physically, mentally, and financially.

My first task was to find what the Government of Canada website had to offer; it had a wealth of information that was difficult to sort through. The list that I had compiled started with the most basic tax benefits for children and went on to more specific aids for those with disabilities. Without too much detail, I worded the information so that it made sense to me:

The **Universal Child Care Benefit (UCCB)** is like a baby shower gift from the government, offering $100 a month for each child that we had under the age of six. We were able to qualify for this benefit because our income was lower, but found out that the amount we received would be taxed annually. Nonetheless, we were able to pay for James' cradle, child seat, and first years' worth of diapers during our first year of enrolment.

> The UCCB is a non-negotiable benefit that every child in Canada that is under the age of 6 receives. This benefit is taxable, so families with higher income that receive this benefit may end up paying back the full amount.

Furthermore, the provincial government of Alberta issued the **Alberta Family Employment Tax Credit (AFETC)** which entitled us to $57 a month to go towards our child until he reached the age of 18. Similarly, Alberta has a program called the **Assured Income for the Severely Handicapped (AISH)**. We are able to receive a monthly living allowance, some health/medical benefits such as prescription drug coverage, optical, and dental, and personal benefits such as infant/child care and education costs, medical equipment, and emergency goods and services.

When we started to focus on how the Canadian government can assist with our child's disability, we found that the **Child Disability Benefit** would pay an amount up to $204.58 per month if we made less than $40,726 yearly. The disability credit begins to be reduced with incomes higher than this. It made our life a little bit easier knowing that a portion of the financial burden of James's disability would be aided by the government. Additionally, as parents of a disabled child, my spouse and I are eligible for the **Disability Tax Credit** which reduces the amount of taxes we pay each year when filing our income tax. The paediatric physician that we were assigned to, following the birth of James, filled out the Disability Tax Credit certificate for us so that we would be able to claim the credit in the following tax year.

Well, this is great information, I thought. But isn't there something more that we can do as parents? What if the government assistance is not enough? What can I do with my

The *Canada Child Tax Benefit* works alongside the UCCB to help families in financial need. It takes into account our yearly income to calculate a monthly payment for each child under the age of 18. A huge relief to us was that unlike the UCCB, this financial aid is not taxed. For a list of Family Tax Credits for low to modest income families in other provinces, please see the section under Provincial Programs.

extra income? And what would happen if we were to pass away while James was still a child?

The last question was the one that bothered me most, but I found the answer easily enough through the Government of Canada website: If the parents of the child were to pass away, the child benefits would be still be available through any legal guardian or caregiver of our child.

My questions started to worry me about James' future. Up until now I had been very diligent about making sure everything in the present was as comfortable as it could be for James, my spouse, and myself, but I hadn't thought of the long term challenges we will have to face as he grew up and also the requirement of a different type of care than what we gave him now. I went to my bank to ask if I could speak to someone about investments. The man I sat down with was a financial adviser and he was able to lead me in the right direction and suggest a plan for my child's future. I told him that I was concerned about James if neither my partner nor I could care for him in the unlikely event of an accident. What the adviser told me was that parents cannot expect to outlive their children, so parents, at any age, should start to plan for their child's continuity of care, especially if the child is disabled. Planning for this as soon as you can will ensure that your child has a comfortable lifestyle when you have passed away.

"Parents cannot expect to outlive their children so they should start to plan for their child's continuity of care... If the parents of the child were to pass away, the child's benefits are still available through the legal guardian or caregiver of the child".

After learning this, I was relieved that I had come in sooner than later. Even if there was no possibility that an accident could occur to me or my spouse, my adviser said it was best to start a plan before any possibility could occur. Additionally, he continued, it was important for us to take advantage of these programs as soon as possible so that we would be able to achieve sizable savings. Many of these programs are available at the start of a disabled child's life.

He introduced us to a savings plan that had just passed legislation in Canada. The **Registered Disability Savings Plan (RDSP)**, he said, had huge potential to give my child a strong financial future. The benefit of this savings program are that any growth (or what is called capital gains) that occurs within the account are completely tax free. In this way, if I was able to find an investment that paid out consistently I would not have to worry about losing any of those earnings to taxes. Not only that, but assuming that we qualify for the account, the government will give James a maximum of $1000 every year, just for having the account open. The $1000 is specific to low-income families such as us. The adviser also said that there are further incentives to putting our own savings into the account. Every year, the Canadian government will put in a maximum of $3500 into James's account if we meet the minimum requirements for depositing our own savings. The minimum deposits we would need to put into the account is $1500 within a one-year period. The maximum contribution of $3500 is obtained because the government triples up to $500 of our deposit. Then, if I deposit from $500 up to $1000, the government will double it. In order for me to maximize the government's contribution, I will need to put $1500 into the RDSP. My first $500 is tripled so the government will give me $1500, and my successive $1000 is doubled to get another $2000 from the government, equalling a total of $3500. The total maximum applies as long as my family has met the financial criteria and the money I invested was within a year. If I wasn't able to put $1500 in for the year, the government will still use the same formula, by tripling the amount until it reaches the $500 threshold, and then doubling any further amounts.

While I was with the adviser, I had not given much thought about the RDSP and it had not made much sense anyway. What I kept thinking about was that I knew we would not be around to care for our son for his full life and it just kept me worrying that he would not make it without us. The adviser convinced me that opening up the RDSP account was a good idea anyway, even if it was just to get $1000. Since we were already eligible for the Disability Tax Credit, it made setting up the RDSP a lot easier. Luckily, we had also applied for a Social Insurance Number for James at birth because we thought it would be important to have when claiming many of the tax deductions. The SIN was another important piece of documentation that we needed to have to set up the RDSP account. The adviser said I would be named the holder on the account, meaning that I manage the account and make decisions about it. I could appoint a joint holder if I feel that I need some assistance in managing the account. For now, I said, I will just have the account open until I had more time to look through the resources and understand them a little better.

"I began to feel a little overwhelmed with all of the financial obligations that I was now faced with keeping track of".

I decided to relax for a few days to calm my nerves and remind myself that I had already discovered a great deal of resources for our finances. When I had reached a more focused and objective state, I looked through the papers I had received from the bank and recalled what the adviser had told me and the savings plan began to make more sense.

If I put some of my savings into the RDSP and bought a well-performing stock that consistently paid out, all of the money I earned from these pay-outs (dividends) would not be taxed because the stock was bought under a registered government plan. Of course, I'm not restricted to buying just stocks. I have the option of buying different investment vehicles (such as bonds, mutual funds, options, and exchange-traded funds) or simply holding the money in a savings account (where the interest wouldn't be taxed) or doing any combination of these strategies. If I invest in the same stock without registering it under the RDSP, the dividend would be taxed as income –same goes for the savings account, the interest would be taxed. The only thing is that the RDSP would belong to my disabled child and I would not be able to use any of the money in the account. Only my child would have access. Looking back to the information package that was given to me, the attractiveness of the account was not really that the dividends or interest wouldn't be taxed, but more so that the government adds $1000 into the account every year that it is open, and can add up to another $3500 yearly if my savings deposits meet the criteria. If I could put $125 into the RDSP each month, then I would reach $1500 at the end of the year and receive $3500 from the government in addition to the $1000 given just for having this account open. That is a potential of $4500 from the government just by contributing $1500.

I began planning for our son's future the moment we had some spare income to invest. However, I knew that I wasn't comfortable enough to make the financial decisions about the RDSP alone, so I decided to appoint my spouse's sister, James's godmother, joint holdership on the RDSP.

Of all the things that a mother dreams about when having a child, one thing that we will never get to experience is our baby's first steps. But James will grow up and he will want to move around and do things by himself, for himself. After our first year, I knew we had to start thinking about our son's future. We had to plan for accessibility because we wanted our son to be strong and confident and he cannot be confident in himself if he couldn't do things independently. We had planned to save some money to start renovating the house as soon as James had reached preschool. So far, we had been fairly successful in putting a little bit of money into James's RDSP each month, even though we didn't always meet the minimum for the additional grant. There was a government of Alberta grant we were able to apply for called **Residential Access Modification Program (RAMP)**. This $5000 grant would help us transform our home to be more wheelchair-accessible for James. We knew that the Child Disability Credit would make it a lot less stressful, but well into the end of the first year it was unknown to us that we could get assistance for basic medical equipment such as his wheel chair without having to spread our already tight budget even further.

If you are not an Alberta resident, the Residential Rehabilitation Assistance Program for Persons with Disabilities (RRAP-D) is another program that offers financial assistance to home modifications for persons with disabilities. This program is funded by the Canada Mortgage and Housing Corporation and all Canadian residents are eligible.
For more information please see Chapter 4.

Another program called **Assured Income for the Severely Handicapped (AISH)** was also available through the Alberta government. This program provided James and our family with a monthly living allowance, which we used to pay a portion of our mortgage and the remainder for home modifications, medical supplies (such as the wheelchair James received) as well as health care and personal benefits. Looking back, I am glad this program existed for residents of Alberta. We depended on this program a lot while James was growing up. As long as James is a resident of Alberta, AISH will be able to offer James support James throughout his lifetime. Some remaining expenses that weren't covered for by the Alberta Government were deducted off our income tax as a **Medical Expense Tax Credit**.

We began to notice a change in James when he was at the age of eight, it seemed that he was not as happy as he once was when he started his first few years of school. It seemed that he was depressed about not being like the other children and was feeling somewhat lost. We tried to talk to him, but he told us we wouldn't understand. It was then that we knew he just wanted other children to talk to, friends that he would not feel judged against or somewhere he could write about his difficulties and feelings. We spoke with our social worker and he suggested *Ability Online*. We were elated to discover that *Ability Online* was a very special website where children with disabilities would be able to chat and interact with other children who are in the same position. We knew this would be great for when we had to take James to his hospital appointments as he would not need to feel isolation when he was stuck in a hospital bed. It didn't take long before he was able to make some fast friends online and was even able to find someone within our city that had a very similar disability in his age group.

For Christmas that year we purchased a laptop for James so that he wouldn't have to come out to the family room to use the computer. He was the only student in his class that had a laptop and that made him feel very special. It was around that time that his classmates began to talk and interact with him more and he began to feel a little bit more a part of the group. Our whole family became involved in Ability Online and we often went on daily to check out any new events, updates, or tips about caring for our disabled son. The website also proved to be a great way for him and us to learn more about activities that were available. We had decided that we would become more involved in the community and not hide in the shadow of our son's disability. This, we hoped, would also teach James that he was capable of doing things just like everyone else and give him a sense of involvement in our community.

"We decided to become more involved in our community... this, we hoped, would teach him that he was capable and give him a sense of involvement".

As James' 10th birthday approached, we thought of a very special gift that we could get him. James was an only child and although he had a few friends on the internet and at his school, we still felt that he was feeling very lonely most of his time. Even though we were involved with the community at bi-weekly events, James didn't like to visit his friends very much because of accessibility. He ended up spending a lot of time at home and doing only a very small variety of things. When his grades started slipping, his teacher said "he was a smart boy that was starting to get bored". We knew that James had great potential and was a very bright kid, so I was not very surprised when boredom was the problem for him not doing so well anymore.

We had turned to the guidance of one of the mentors we were close with on *Ability Online*. She had suggested that the responsibility and challenge of taking care of a pet would be a good idea. Her experience came from her own son, who had become nearly paralyzed after a car accident. Her son was a lot older than James and having his life transform in the middle of his youth really took a toll on his outlook on life... that was until they were introduced to a therapy dog that came to visit every weekend at the rehabilitation centre. The dog and her boy really bonded and when the rehabilitation was complete, they knew it would take more than their support to keep their son going.

So we set out to contact some very special dog trainers. One of them worked with a society called *Dogs With Wings,* an assistance society who specialized in the training of assistance dogs. We had a visit with the training center and some of the puppies that were being trained and we decided to fill out the paperwork and make an appointment for a few more meetings to find a successful match. James was ecstatic when we introduced him to his future pet. For the first time in many months his eyes lit up and he busied himself in planning for the arrival of his friend, making sure that there were enough comfy places for the dog to sleep, deciding where the food and water bowl would be kept, and the best places to go for walks. For James, this was a blessing. He began to enjoy his time more and I knew he felt he had a responsibility towards his dog. James's dog, Buster, helped James by balancing him as he moved from place to place. He also knew how to retrieve objects that were out-of-reach for James, or objects that had fallen into a nook. As days turned into weeks, we noticed that James had gained more confidence in himself and became more independent. Many of the daily challenges that I had to help James with were now accomplished by Buster and I knew James felt more comfortable with the dog helping his disability rather than his mother. Our boy was starting to grow up and felt embarrassed that his parents wanted to monitor his every action, so as Buster and James grew closer, we trusted Buster as James' guide to walk him to school. It was only a few blocks away from where we lived and the dog got a special seat beside James during his classes. When school was finished, we would pick them up and usually head to the dog park where Buster could let loose and be a dog again.

Buster remained as James' best friend for the very important chapters of James' life as he grew up, joined his first sports team in junior high school, excelled in his debate team throughout high school, and was granted a scholarship for entry into university overseas. We had financially prepared for this moment, but emotionally there was no way. We maximized the RDSP by putting money into it whenever we could and at the age of 18, James had over $100,000 to spend to whatever costs he needed to face in the future. But the fact that James would be overseas pursuing his dreams and that we would not be able to be by his side troubled us very deeply. Buster was old and semi-retired now and James did not want any other dog. There was no way he would be able to take Buster along.

We knew we had to let James grasp this valuable opportunity to study overseas. We didn't want to hold him back due to fear, and our own insecurities about his condition. So the summer months leading to his departure we contacted the disabilities agency in the city of his stay and made arrangements with them to meet near the beginning of the school year. I accompanied James to his home for the next 6 months and we met with the disability support personnel in this city of residence as well as the disability support staff at his school. For the first week of school I rented a room in a hotel not far from his dorm and made sure there were no unforeseen issues. Surprisingly, everything went more smoothly than I could have possibly imagined. Many tears were shed when the final day had come, even though James had reassured me again and again he would be fine. With great reluctance I left, reminding myself that I would not be there for James forever, and that this was the first and very necessary step to take to help him improve his own life.

James is now in his final year of his political science degree. He has been to four different countries and nine different cities worldwide since he left Alberta to pursue his studies. We visit whenever we can and are always here to offer support, even from afar. As the end of the school year approaches, I know that James will be successful in all of his life endeavours. As I look back on his life growing up, I am glad myself and my husband took the steps necessary to ensure his safety and security, and to develop his confidence and independence. When I look back there is not a thing I regret.

For most mothers, taking care of a newborn baby is a struggle in itself. New mothers are overloaded with information about how to care for their child and what abnormalities to look out for during the pregnancy and after birth. Now imagine the amount of information a mother that is pregnant with a disabled child would receive during her months of pregnancy.

Being the caregiver of a child is a full-time job. Being the caregiver of a disabled child is a full-time job with a lifetime of dedication. The struggles and decisions that mothers and caregivers of disabled children must face are very complex. They must strive to achieve the balance between providing care and protection without taking away freedom and independence. They must balance the time they spend managing the child's illness or disability and the time they spend with child. And there is a constant struggle between how much to put away for the future and how much needs to be spent at present to give the child a comfortable standard of living.

We have outlined some of the key topics in this chapter for you to consider and to begin a strategy that may help you overcome these decisions. You will also find descriptions of each of the programs provided by the Canadian Government to give you an idea of the type of help you may receive.

☑ **Universal Child Care Benefit:** Automatic application occurs when the mother of the newborn registers the birth of the child and gives consent on the provincial or territorial birth registration form.

☑ **Canada Child Tax Benefit and National Child Benefit Supplement:** Automatic application occurs the same way as the Universal Child Care Benefit. If you did not apply using this method, please see the sections below on how to apply for the benefits above.

☑ **Child Disability Benefit:** Application of this benefit must occur simultaneously with the application of the Canada Child Tax Benefit or after enrolment in the CCTB. The T2201, Disability Tax Credit Certificate must be filled out and mailed to a tax centre stated on the form.

☑ **Disability Tax Credit:** Enrolment into this tax credit occurs after completion and submission of the T2201, Disability Tax Credit Certificate

☑ **Medical Expense Tax Credit:** Enrolment into this tax credit occurs after completion and submission of the T2201, Disability Tax Credit Certificate

☑ **Canadian Pension Plan Child Benefits:** Application kits may be found online by searching http://www.servicecanada.gc.ca/ for CPP, obtaining the kit from a Service Canada Centre and many funeral homes, or by calling 1-800-277-9914 TTY: 1-800-255-4786

☑ **Registered Disability Savings Plan**: Applications are made through your local bank or financial institution. The applicant must be approved for the Disability Tax Credit to be approved for this savings plan.

☑ **Canada Learning Bond:** Applications are made through your local bank or financial institution. The applicant must be approved for the National Child Benefit Supplement.

☑ **Children's Arts Tax Credit and Children's Fitness Amount:** The Children's Fitness Amount may be claimed on Line 365 of your tax return. The Children's Arts Tax credit can be claimed in 2011 and subsequent tax years' Schedule 1 Federal Tax form.

Resources

Federal/National Programs:

Universal Child Care Benefit (UCCB)

The UCCB provides a $100 payment for each child that is under the age of six. The payment is taxable which means that when you file a tax return the $100 is considered a part of your earned income. You are not required to file a tax return to receive the UCCB, automatic application occurs when the mother of the newborn registers the birth of the newborn with the province or territory. Only the mother is able to sign a consent form (the Automatic Benefits Application) to apply to this program during the registration of her newborn. The Canada Revenue Agency will then determine eligibility. You are eligible to apply to the program as soon as your child is born, if your child is under the age of six, or if you/your spouse or common law partner has a child who is six years of age and one of you becomes eligible (i.e. a Canadian citizen, permanent resident, protected person, or temporary resident).

However, if you are not currently receiving the UCCB and you are the person primarily responsible for the care and upbringing of the child, then you may apply for this benefit as well as the Canada Child Tax Benefit (listed below) and any related provincial or territorial programs using the Automated Benefits Application (APA) or the Canada Child Benefits Application. Do not reapply if you have given consent on the provincial or territorial birth registration form. This will only delay processing or payment issuing.

The APA is presently only running in Quebec, Prince Edward Island, Nova Scotia, Ontario, and British Columbia, however other provinces and territories will be adapting this service in the near future. Please see http://www.cra-arc.gc.ca/bnfts/tmtd_ prv-eng.html on how to use this feature if your child is a resident of one of the above provinces.

The Canada Child Benefits application form may be accessed at http://www.cra-arc.gc.ca/E/pbg/tf/rc66/README.html Otherwise, you may contact your local tax center, or call the Canadian Revenue Agency at 1-800-387-1193

Canada Child Tax Benefit (CCTB)

There are several tax incentives that are available not only for disabled children but for any child. The largest one from the Canadian government pays a monthly non-taxable amount to help eligible families with the cost of raising children under 18 years of age. Eligible families are selected based on financial need and this is assessed when taxes are filed. The benefit amount received is calculated based on the family net income, which excludes the amount received from the UCCB. However, if you have to repay the UCCB, this portion is included in your family net income calculation. The benefit is calculated in July for the previous year, so even if you think you may not qualify due to high income, you should still apply.

The CCTB is accessible to the family as soon as your child is born; or a child starts to live with you; or you become a resident of Canada, with either of the requirements met. The following criteria must be met to qualify for this payment: you must live with the child, the child must be under the age of 18, you must be the person who is mainly caring for and raising the child; Which means you are responsible for watching over the child's daily activities and needs, making sure the child's medical needs are met, and arranging for child care when necessary—you do

CCTB

Number of Children	Basic CCTB	NCBS	Total	Monthly Benefit
1st child	$1255	$1945	$3200	$266.67
2nd child	$1255	$1720	$2975	$247.92
each additional child	$1343	$1637	$2980	$248.33

Number of children for whom you receive the CCTB	Base amount
1	$40,970
2	$40,968
3	$40,954
4	$46,234
5	$51,513
6	$56,792
7	$62,071
8	$67,251
9 or more	Contact the CRA

not need to be the parent of this child to receive this benefit, however, you (regardless if you are married or single) or your spouse or common-law partner must be a Canadian citizen, a permanent resident, a protected person, or a temporary resident who has lived in Canada for the past 18 months, and who has a valid permit during the 19th month. To apply for the Canada Child Tax Benefit, visit the Canadian Revenue Agency website, or contact them. Both can be found in the Index of this book.

The CCTB may include the National Child Benefit Supplement and the Child Disability Benefit. The CCTB will also include provincial tax credits issued to families with low- to moderate-income that have children under the age of 18.

Starting in July 2011 one lump-sum payment of the CCTB will be paid to families that receive less than $20 per month. This one-time payment will cover the entire benefit year from July 2011 to June 2012.

National Child Benefit Supplement (NCBS):

This is an additional program that is included in the CCTB and paid monthly to low-income families with children under 18 years of age. The supplement is the Government of Canada's contribution to the National Child Benefit (NCB). As part of the NCB, certain provinces and territories also provide complementary benefits and services for children in low-income families, such as child benefits, earned income supplements, and supplementary health benefits, as well as child care, children-at-risk, and early childhood services.

For more information, visit the NCB web site:
http://nationalchildbenefit.ca.

The following information is adapted from this website:

• Families with net incomes below $20,435 will get the maximum CCTB - including the full NCBS and the supplement for the third and each additional child - of:
- • $266.67 per month ($3,200 per year) for the first child,
- • $247.92 per month ($2,975 per year) for the second child, and
- • $248.33 per month ($2,980 per year) for all other children in the family, along with any supplement for children under 7 that is applicable.

• Families with net incomes between $20,435 and $36,378 will get the maximum basic CTB, the supplement for the third and each additional child, and a partial NCBS, along with any supplement for children under 7 that is applicable. Families with four or more children will also be entitled to a partial NCBS if their income is just above $36,378.

• One and two-child families with net incomes between $36,378 and approximately $99,128 will receive partial benefits. Larger families may also be entitled to a partial CCTB if their income is above $99,128.

• The annual Children's Special Allowances amount will increase from $2,949.96 to $3,200.04. The monthly amount per child will increase from $245.83 to $266.67 in July 2006.

Child Disability Benefit (CDB):

This is a disability benefit paid monthly to families of disabled children under the age of 18 who are eligible for the CCTB. If the CCTB has not yet been applied for, you must also complete this benefit form and mail it to your tax centre. The CDB entitles the family to a maximum of $205.83 per month for each disabled child. The amount that each disabled child receives will be included in the CCTB and is based on the family income after taxes. Unlike the CCTB, the money received on this benefit is not subject to tax. The individual or a legal representative must fill out part A of the T2201, Disability Tax Credit Certificate and a qualified practitioner (i.e. family doctor) must fill out Part B for the individual to apply for this benefit. This form may be filled out at any time and the completed form has a list of addresses of tax centres that it may be mailed to. If you are approved for the CDB, the amount you receive will be calculated for the current and two previous CCTB years; for years beyond these, a written request forwarded to the tax centre or tax services office must be submitted.

For more information and eligibility, visit the CRA's CDB website:
http://www.cra-arc.gc.ca/bnfts/dsblty-eng.html
The information below is adapted from this website.

For the period of July 2010 to June 2011, the CDB provided up to $2,470 per year ($205.83 per month) for each child who is eligible for the disability amount.

The CDB amount is calculated using a base amount, which is associated with the number of children for whom you receive the CCTB. You will receive the full CDB amount if your adjusted family net income[1] is **less** than the base amount for your family size, as indicated in the chart.

If your adjusted family net income is more than the base amount, you will receive a lower amount of CDB. The amount will be

---

1   The income that your family earns after taxes but excludes any money you receive from the Universal Child Care Benefit (UCCB). However, if you have received too much UCCB the amount you paid back will be included as part of your adjusted family net income.

Number of Children for whom you receive the CCTB	Base Amount
1	$41,544
2	$41,536
3	$41,520
4	$46,871
5	$52,222
6	$57,574
7	$62,925
8	$68,276
9 or more	Contact the CRA

reduced as follows:
- If you have one child who is eligible for the CDB, the amount of CDB is reduced by 2% of your adjusted family net income that is more than the base amount for one child (see the above chart).
- If you have two or more children who are eligible for the CDB, the amount of CDB is reduced by 4% of your adjusted family net income that is more than the base amount for the number of children for which you receive the CDB (see the above chart).

Disability Tax Credit

A tax deduction that can be claimed for yourself, if you are disabled, or be transferred from a disabled dependent to the caregiver (in this case, from a disabled child to either parent or guardian). First, a qualified medical practitioner, such as a family doctor, must assess the disabled individual and certify that there is a severe and prolonged impairment under certain guidelines:

- He or she is blind.
- He or she is markedly restricted in any one of the following basic activities of daily living:
  - speaking;
  - walking;
  - dressing; or
  - elimination (bowel or bladder functions);
  - hearing;
  - feeding;
  - performing the mental functions necessary for everyday life

- He or she needs, and must dedicate a certain amount of time specifically for, life-sustaining therapy to support a vital function

The tax form <u>T2201, Disability Tax Credit Certificate</u> is needed for the certification process. Once the form is completed you need to address it to the Disability Tax Credit Unit of the tax centre; the addresses are indicated on the form itself. The credit is then granted to you as a reduction on your income taxes.

IMPORTANT: If you are denied for the disability tax credit it is possible and highly encouraged that you appeal the ruling. The Canada Revenue Agency has recently made it more difficult to be accepted into the program due to the increased benefit of the Registered Disability Savings Plan. It is in your best interest to appeal if you are turned down as there is no harm or loss of benefit to re-apply and upon receiving this tax credit, other disability benefits and programs become accessible to you.

Medical Expense Tax Credit

A tax deduction that can be claimed for yourself or your dependents on total eligible medical expenses incurred in the year. The amount of money incurred throughout the year on medical expenses or devices can be claimed on Line 330 or Line

331 of your tax return. The subtle difference between which line of your tax return you should claim under lies in the year of birth of the child you are claiming from. If the dependent child is born in 1993 or later, use Line 330. If the dependent child is born in 1992 or earlier, use Line 331. To be eligible to claim this tax credit, a qualified practitioner must certify the form T2201, Disability Tax Credit Certificate. Eligible medical expenses include many assistance materials for the blind, deaf, or immobile.

For a list of items that may be credited and the certification that may be required for certain items, see:
http://www.cra-arc.gc.ca/tx/ndvdls/tpcs/ncm-tx/rtrn/cmpltng/ddctns/lns300-350/330/llwbl-eng.html

IMPORTANT: For the 2011 tax year, medical expenses incurred for an eligible dependent are no longer restricted to $10,000 per year. If you had spent over this amount in 2010, you may be able to claim the remainder as long as the purchase falls within a 12-month time period. For instance, if $15,000 was spent on medical expenses from July 2010 until April 2011 and only $10,000 was claimed on your 2010 tax return, $5000 tax credit can be put towards a tax credit between the period of January 2011 to July 2011.

Canadian Pension Plan (CPP) Children Benefits

If a CPP contributor is disabled or deceased, a monthly benefit can be paid to the dependent natural or adopted children of the contributor(s) or a child in the care and control of a CPP contributor. Children that have turned 25 are no longer eligible for these benefits. Children between the ages of 18 to 24 must be attending school full time to receive the benefit. Children under the age of 18 do not have to be in school to be eligible. An application should be made as soon as the CPP contributor has applied for a disability benefit or has passed away because the benefit can only make back payments up to 11 months from the time the application was received. Two separate benefits may be received if both parents or guardians paid in to the CPP and each parent or guardian is either deceased or receiving the CPP disability benefit. The average monthly CPP benefit paid, in the case of a disability is $214.85 (amount from September 2010 data); the maximum monthly CPP benefit paid is $218.50 (2011). Children of deceased contributors average monthly payment is $214.85 (from September 2010 data) and maximum monthly payment is $218.50 (2011).

For more information visit:
http://www.servicecanada.gc.ca/eng/isp/pub/factsheets/studben.shtml

A link to an application form is found on the web address above as well. Otherwise an Application Kit with instructions is available from any Service Canada Centre and many funeral homes. You may also ask for a free kit or assistance by calling **1-800-277-9914** TTY: **1-800-255-4786**

Registered Disability Savings Plan

One of the best ways that you can prepare for what's ahead is to have an RDSP set up for your child so that you may qualify for a yearly $1000 grant from the federal government. Another benefit of this type of investment is that interest gained within this investment is not subject to being taxed. Tax-deferred savings means that any growth that accumulates in the account will not be subject to tax until it is taken out of the RDSP to be used. The reason you want to begin saving and planning for your child's needs after you have passed is due to compounding.

Some financial institutions may charge fees when setting up an RDSP. Such fees may include administration, set-up, and management fees. Additionally, if you choose to move your RDSP from one financial institution to another, you will be charged a fee ranging from $25-$50.

Specified Disability Savings Plan (SDSP)
For those with shortened life expectancy

As of 2011 it is now possible to withdraw the government grant from the RDSP without having to wait 10 years. This applies to individuals with shortened life expectancy and medical evidence to support the claim. If the individual's situation improves it is possible that he or she will be able to return the SDSP to an RDSP. Once switched to an SDSP, no deposits are allowed to be contributed and the maximum amount that is allowed to be withdrawn each year is $10,000 of government deposits.

Canada Learning Bond (CLB)

A $500 bond is contributed into a Registered Education Savings Plan (RESP) for a child that is receiving the National Child Benefit Supplement. Children receive an additional $100 bond instalments paid each year that they are eligible for the NCBS up to the age of 15. Up to $2000 plus interest can be used towards your child's post-secondary education. The child must be a beneficiary under an RESP, have a Social Insurance Number and Birth Certificate, and be born on or after January 1, 2004. You can open an RESP for your child through your local bank or financial institution. A small fee may be charged to open this account, but the first $500 bond payment of the CLB will include an extra $25 to cover this cost.

For more information you can visit a Service Canada Centre near you, call **1-800-622-6232**, or visit:
http://www.canlearn.ca/eng/saving/clb/index.shtml

Registered Education Savings Plan and Canada Education Savings Grant

These are additional programs that you can contribute towards to help you save for your child's post-secondary education. We will not be covering these in detail, however, they are great resources for your child's savings if your income is above the eligibility requirements of the programs mentioned above or if you have extra savings that you would like to be put into a tax-deductible plan for your child's continued education.

Children's Fitness and Children's Arts Tax Credit

These tax credits are also eligible for children that are not receiving the disability tax credit, however for the purposes of this book, we will only mention the details for children eligible under the disability tax credit.

These tax credits are based on eligible expenses paid for the cost of registration or membership of a child in a prescribed of artistic, cultural, recreational, or developmental activity. Eligible expenses of up to $500 each year for each of your children under the age of 18 who receive the disability tax credit. If at least $100 has been spent for a child who receives the disability tax credit, an additional $500 can be claimed. The CATC can be claimed for the 2011 and subsequent tax years. If the fees are considered an eligible expense for both the Fitness and Arts Tax Credits, you will not be able to claim the CATC.

For more information and lists of eligible expenses please visit: http://www.cra-arc.gc.ca/tx/ndvdls/tpcs/ncm-tx/rtrn/cmpltng/ddctns/lns360-390/365/menu-eng.html and http://www.cra-arc.gc.ca/gncy/bdgt/2011/qa01-eng.html

Child Special Allowances (CSA)
for all children under 18

The Canada Revenue Agency administers the Children's Special Allowances Act (CSA Act). This allowance is a tax free monthly payment for any child who is under the age of 18, lives in Canada and is looked after by an Agency. Even if a child is still in school once they reach the age of 18, the CSA will no longer be paid.

An Agency is a a federal, provincial, or territorial government department appointed to administer law for the protection and care of children, a group foster home or institution; or an institution licensed or otherwise approved by a province or territory to have the custody and care of children. To be "maintained by an agency" means that the child needs to be cared for by the agency, and is dependent on them for his/her education, training, and advancement to a greater extent than on any other agency.

This does not apply to the majority of people who have children but it is a valuable resource for institutions like foster homes.

Provincial Programs

Alberta Family Employment Tax Credit (AFETC)

The AFETC is a non-taxable amount paid to families with working income that have children who are under 18 years of age. You may be entitled to receive: $696 ($58.00 per month) for the first child; $633 ($52.75 per month) for the second child; $380 ($31.66 per month) for the third child; and $127 ($10.58 per month) for the fourth child. The maximum you can get is the lesser of $1,836 and 8% of your family's working income that is more than $2,760.The credit is reduced by 4% of the amount of the adjusted family net income that is more than $33,974. Payments are made in July 2011 and January 2012.

This program is fully funded by the Province of Alberta. For more information, call **1-800-959-2809**.

Assured Income for the Severely Handicapped (AISH)

AISH provides a maximum monthly living allowance of $1,588 to assist with living expenses. It is possible to work and receive the AISH benefit. If you are single and make $800 or less in net income per month then you receive the full AISH benefit. Monthly net income amounts above $800 reduce your monthly AISH benefit up to $1. The family AISH benefit also entitles the family $1,588 per month. However, to receive the maximum AISH benefit for a family, the family monthly net income amount must be $1,940 or below. For an up-to-date, detailed guide of this information, please visit http://www.seniors.alberta.ca/aish/tipsheets/EmploymentIncome.pdf

AISH also provides health benefits for prescription drugs, diabetic supplies, optical, dental, emergency ambulance services and an exemption from the Alberta Aids to Daily Living co-pay fees.

More information about his program is available at:
http://www.seniors.alberta.ca/aish
or call the Alberta Supports Contact Centre at:
1-877-644-9992.

Alberta Works

Alberta Works is an income support program for individuals or families. You do not need to be disabled to apply for this. This program is sponsored by the Government of Alberta for low-income individuals who do not have the means to meet basic needs, like food, clothing, and shelter. The level of support will depend on each individual's situation, which includes financial situation, ability to work and the number of children in the family. (Note: The National Child Benefit Supplement is included in the monthly sum that would be paid out to the family.)

Eligibility falls under three categories:

- *Not Expected to Work:* You have difficulty working because of a chronic mental or physical health problem or because of multiple barriers to employment

- *Expected to Work:* You are looking for work, working, or unable to work in the short-term

- *Learners:* You need upgrading or training so you can get a job

Eligible learners can receive up to $5,000 per academic year for training, books, supplies, and living allowance while they are working part time. The earned income from work will not affect the dollar amount received per academic year.

Those who are eligible for Income Support also receive:
- health benefits for themselves and their dependants
- information and training to find a job
- help to obtain child support payments

For more information, visit:
http://employment.alberta.ca/albertaworks/
If you are a resident of Alberta, dial **310-0000** for toll-free, province-wide access.

Residential Access Modification Program (RAMP)

A grant of up to $5,000 is sponsored by the Alberta Government for eligible wheelchair users to modify their home to become more wheelchair-accessible. Applicant households must have an annual income of $36,900 or less.

This maximum annual income is increased for each of the following situations:
- $9,600 for addition of a spouse (i.e. combined annual income is $46,500 or less)
- $9,600 for each child under 21 year of age, living at home and attending school full-time
- $7,131 for each child under the age of 18 who is living at home and also using a wheelchair

Criteria for eligibility are outlined below:
- All wheelchair users, regardless of age, within program guidelines (homeowner, tenants, and natives living on and off reserve, persons living with family)

- Canadian citizens or permanent residents
- Aboriginal people living off- and on-reserve
- People with neuro-degenerative diseases (multiple sclerosis; muscular dystrophy; ALS [Lou Gehrig's disease]; COPD [chronic obstructive pulmonary disease]; non-recovering stroke victim; Parkinson's disease; Alzheimer's disease; spina bifida; spinal cord injuries)
- Seniors aged 75+ and considered medically frail (those using a walker)
- Only one wheelchair user per household may apply for assistance, in most cases

You do not need to own the house you want to modify. If you are renting, the landlord needs to fill out the Property Modification Approval form in the tenant application package for permanent modifications. The landlord can also approve temporary modifications with this form. If you've made modifications without applying, reimbursements can be made by applying within the first 90 days after completion of modifications. Applications after the 90 days period, but within one year, are reviewed on a case-by-case basis. Applicants are expected to live at their current address for 5 years after the modifications have been completed.

For more information and application packages, visit: http://www.seniors.alberta.ca/aadl/ramp/
You may also call **1-877-427-5760** or E-mail RAMP@gov.ab.ca

Other Provincial* Family Tax Credits for low- to moderate-income families with children under the age of 18**:

- B.C. Family Bonus Program (includes Basic Family Bonus and the B.C. Earned Income Benefit)
- Saskatchewan Low-Income Tax Credit
- Ontario Child Benefit Quebec – applications for child assistance programs must be filed with the Régie des rentes du Québec
- Nova Scotia Child Benefit and the Nova Scotia Affordable Living Tax Credit
- New Brunswick Child Tax Benefit
- Newfoundland and Labrador Child Benefit and Mother Baby Nutrition Supplement and Newfoundland and Labrador Harmonized Sales Tax Credit

...

*The Canada Revenue Agency does not administer any benefit programs on behalf of Manitoba or Prince Edward Island

**The Newfoundland and Labrador Harmonized Sales Tax Credit will apply to each child under 19 years of age

Other Helpful Resources:

PLAN (http://plan.ca)
This website is for those families with a disabled child or relative that have the question "Who will take care of them when we are gone?"

PLAN's mission is to help families secure the future for their relative with a disability and to provide peace of mind. This website allows families and individuals to sign up as members that receive support through other members, subscriptions to information affecting families with someone that has a disability, and a network of other resources to help you understand more about taking care of an individual with a disability.

If all of these disability applications still seem daunting, the good news is that there are people to help.

The **Ability Tax Group** (http://abilitytax.ca/) are a group of professionals who will help ensure that you receive as much help as possible from the government and will show you what options there are available in terms of government assistance. They will help you apply to receive the Disability Tax Credit and open your Registered Disability Savings Plan. Their website also offers an introduction to Trust and Estate planning, which we cover in chapter 5. Log on to their website for a free online assessment or you can call them at **1-877-690-0330**.

having an adult child

with disabilities

Chapter 3

Chapter 3
Having an Adult Child with Disabilities

Before the accident I had thought that I was going to live out a "normal" life as I had the previous 20 years. In the wake of my disability, I realized that I would have to change my whole life, my habits, and learn to adapt.

Shortly after I had completed my first year of university I was diagnosed with a severe disability after a snowboarding accident that had damaged some of my brain functions. During the first stages of my recovery I thought that my disability would be temporary, that I would improve, and that I would be able to carry on as usual. But as the rehabilitation went on, further diagnoses suggested that the damage was likely to be permanent and life-long. I was going to be disabled for the rest of my life and I was only 22. Even with that being the case, I had never lost sight of trying to put my life back together.

To my parents' credit, they tried to be strong and be there for me in every way possible. But it was especially difficult for my mom; she had difficulties dealing with our new reality. First, was the shock that I could not perform simple everyday tasks, like getting myself a cup of water without spilling or dropping the cup. Second, was the fact that I would not be able to continue with university at this point in my life. My life focus had shifted to getting my disability under control—I had to drop out of university during my second year. My parents were very supportive of me even if they couldn't face the reality of my illness, but if it had not been for their support I do not think I would have been able to come to terms with my new limitations. My parents' perceptions also seemed to change once I was diagnosed—they became very protective of me.

> *"Activities I had once enjoyed were no longer a part of my life. I gave them up because I simply could not do it anymore".*

I knew that the only way I would be able to get better and become functional was to continue to focus on my therapy. But, I discovered that my therapy would last for many, many months, and there was no way that I could do anything other than try to regain day-to-day functions. I could no longer ride my bike anymore, I could not stand or read for very long periods of time, I couldn't even go out for very long unattended because walking around would leave me exhausted. Activities I had once enjoyed were no longer a part of my life. I gave them up because I simply could not do it anymore.

Insurance companies will cover expenses for dependent overage children if you have coverage at the time of the accident. Most require that the dependent child over the age of 18 must attend a post-secondary institution. National banks offer insurance as well as many other insurance companies. If your employer does not offer insurance through a group plan, you may contact these insurance companies to purchase private coverage for yourself and your family.

One of the only things that made me feel better was that I could still purchase items that I wanted and spend a little money on an occasional short outing. There was no way I would be able to be employed at this time in my current mentally and physically diminished state and I didn't think I would be able to find a job very easily because of it. I began to feel useless and my previous goals of financial freedom became unachievable as I was only able to spend what my parents were giving me and a small amount that I would receive from their insurance company. The only reason that I was covered under insurance was due to being in school when the accident happened; I was considered a dependent-student at that time under my parents' plan. The insurance income was incredibly fortunate for me as I still wanted to be able to enjoy my life as fully as possible, but more importantly, I had to work around my disability somehow.

Spending freely had become more troublesome, with very little left after the medication and rehabilitation costs were covered. My parents suffered a huge financial setback after the accident, paying for all the costs incurred. They were just managing to stay out of debt when they found a special program for those with lower income; **Ontario Works** supports families with lower income when a family member has a substantial physical or mental disability. The monthly amount varies by the family income, assets, housing costs, and size of family. Since I was already enrolled in receiving monthly aid from the **Canadian Pension Plan**, this affected the amount our family was able to obtain from Ontario's Income Support. Nevertheless, Ontario's provincial program made my life somewhat easier as the pressure and guilt of being dependent on my parents lifted.

Any individual that is 18 and over and has been or is currently employed has made contributions to the Canadian Pension Plan. Certain criteria allow these contributions to be withdrawn for disability payments.

It had not been long, thankfully, until I had discovered the **Registered Disability Savings Plan** through my bank. When I met a financial adviser to discuss how to balance my income with my expenses, she told me that I could actually receive up to $1,000 per year from the Canadian Government just for opening up an account called the Registered Disability Savings Plan (RDSP). She also told me that I could potentially gain another $3,500 per year from the Government if I put some

To apply for an RDSP, the beneficiary must be eligible for the Disability Tax Credit. It takes 90 days for the $1000 grant to be deposited into the account, but this grant must remain in the account for 10 years. Other government contributions follow this rule as well until the plan holder reaches 61 years of age. Certain exceptions apply. See below for details.

money into the account. The only catch is that the money from the government is not accessible immediately. Each government contribution will have to remain in my registered savings plan for 10 years until I can put it to use. This was a great opportunity for me to invest in the future so I opened up an account; however, I told her I could not afford the extra deposits at this point. To my surprise, she told me that friends or family could contribute on my behalf and that it's a great thing to keep in mind once I adjusted to my situation a little.

Even with all the difficulties my parents were going through with me I maintained my interest in doing all of the activities that I used to. But, my parents were protective and would try to dissuade me from going out to party, or even simple things like taking the bus to get to places. It was beginning to happen more and more often as I began to regain some control of my body. I felt like I was ready to take my life back but as I pushed for more freedom with my regained abilities my parents' became more protective, so much so that I couldn't leave the house without them asking where I was going and what I was going out to do. Many arguments arose from these situations. I was an adult and that they shouldn't try to treat me as a child, even if I was disabled. I told them I wanted to live my life my way, and that they wouldn't be able to stop me. I was so incredibly frustrated at my independence being taken away that I began looking for any chance to get away from my parents to gain some freedom. I knew they were just trying to help me, but they didn't seem to understand that I didn't want to see myself as someone who was disabled so badly I had to depend on others. I wanted to be treated like I had before. To be treated like someone who is disabled, but not dependent.

My plan was to get a simple rental property, but this was difficult as I was still unemployed and I would not be able to afford the rent, food, utilities and my weekly visits to my therapy sessions. Along with regular visits to different doctors, getting my disability under control had become a full time job. There was a ton of paperwork I had to constantly keep up with to insure I was covered under private and public health. For many months I felt very hopeless as the majority of my life was being sunk into trying to get "better" so that I could become independent even though I knew I would never be at the same level as I had been before. It was taking a long time and I didn't notice any new improvements. I knew I had to make a change for my life to progress. The change that I chose was to leave my parents' home and the people who had looked after me and had been there for me whenever I needed anything. But what I needed even more so was to get away so I could do things for myself again.

I spoke to my therapist and she told me that they had determined that I was rehabilitated enough to perform day-to-day tasks without supervision as long as I continued to arrive for therapy. After learning the good news, I went my social worker at the clinic and she suggested that I look into going into **Non-Profit or Co-Op Housing**. I am told that the city of Ottawa can provide subsidies and the majority of the eligible renters pay no more than 30% of their income in a variety of domiciles such as high rise and low rise condos, townhouses, rooming houses, and units for people with special needs or disabilities. The subsidized housing would allow me to adapt to living on my own

You must contact a co-ordinated access centre to apply for Ontario's Non-Profit or Co-Op Housing, or you may apply directly at a local non-profit housing area. Subsidies from the Ontario government are applied for at the same time and the more buildings you apply for, the faster it will take for you to move up the waiting list.

at an affordable rate and it was close to a support centre that would offer me aide when and if I needed it. The only downside was that the waiting lists for Non-Profit Housing are incredibly long. In the larger municipalities of Ontario families can wait up to ten years.

> *"The residents seemed like a close-knit community that helped each other... they were a diverse group of people who respected one-another".*

I was wary at first about going into an area where all families there depended on subsidized housing. I didn't have any idea what the people would be like. Would the residents be disabled or different in any way? But I wanted out of my parent's basement and wanted freedom so I took her up on this offer. She showed me to a couple of the subsidized homes in the city, they all seemed well maintained and kept, and the people that I met there were all very friendly. There were families with children, seniors, and people like me with special needs. The residents seemed like a very close-knit community that helped each other out whenever they could. I felt more comfortable knowing that it was a very diverse group of people that lived in these communities who respected one-another because we were all independent individuals with one thing in common—we just needed a little bit of help finding affordable living. We applied for subsidized housing in several different areas to increase my chances.

My social worker also told me that I was eligible for an annual bus pass for the reduced cost of $45, since I was on disability and social assistance. This was great because I am no longer able to operate a car, but it would allow me to have an increased level of freedom and a handy way for me to get from place-to-place. It would be another couple of years before I was finally able to get into a subsidized rental property that was about an hour away from where I used to live, so the bus pass was something that I definitely couldn't live without.

One night, while in my parents' basement, I was lamenting about how I wanted to get into the work force. The financial situation was still tight and it took just about everything I had to live my new independent lifestyle. One of the service staff suggested that I speak with the Ministry of Community and Social Services as they helped all disabled people with training to get into the workforce. This was a great opportunity for me.

The Opportunities Fund for Persons with Disabilities is a federal program that can help you prepare for, obtain, and maintain employment or self-employment. It is directed to people who are not eligible for Employment Insurance benefits and sponsors activities that will help you get into the workforce by working with you and your own business or employers. For more information, please see this topic below.

Since I was already receiving **Ontario Disability Income Support,** I didn't need to fill out an application for **Ontario's Employment Support program**. This program helped me find a job and assisted in the training of my new job. The staff linked me with a service provider which helped me develop my career goals and an action plan to achieve it. They were able to find me a job that was convenient for public transit to transport me from the Co-Op home to work. My first day back in the workforce and my first day in my new home were so closed together that I was overwhelmed with a sense of accomplishment. Even now, I knew that was a pivotal point in my life which helped me flourish as an individual. It may not have been the job that I was going to university for but I was getting my life back on track and dealing with my disability one step at a time.

Eventually after working for a couple of years with the company, I wanted to leave the subsidized home and live on my own. My social worker was really great in helping me get all of my things together. I was able to contact the employment support program to get funding for me to move into my new place, as it was even closer and more convenient for me to get to work. I also got my parents involved as I wanted to move closer to them on the condition that they would be there to support me, not to look after me like a child. That was my one and only condition, and I know it sounds silly to have a condition on your parents help but to feel useful I had to feel independent.

I was able to work full-time but purchasing a home immediately was unnecessary and costly, however, it was definitely a part of my long-term goals. I decided a rent-to-own property would be ideal, and luckily, a few new condos were being built around the area that I was interested in. Having just turned 28 and having been with my disability for the last 5 years, I was more knowledgeable about housing than I had been when I had first moved out. I knew that I could apply for special loan provisions through **Canada Mortgage & Housing Corporation (CMHC)** to support a modified living space suited to my disability. After signing an agreement to purchase, I inquired at the condo office immediately so that the builders of the condo could perform the proper upgrades to my new home with a greatly reduced cost. In about 5 months I would finally be able to achieve the amount of freedom I had hoped for.

Many years later, I had found some stability in life. I continued to pay off my condo and I had a great job that would earn enough income for me to feel secure; most importantly I had my disability under control. I looked back on my struggles and I realized I was able to accomplish a lot, and with the right support team, I was able and am capable of doing a lot of things independently. Not many disabled people can say this, but I felt really accomplished and amazingly I felt like I needed a new challenge to overcome. I decided that I was going to finish my university degree and went to look into support programs for my education.

My current expenses were under control and I had only started to save a little bit of money for my education—most of my previous savings had been put into the RDSP. I knew that I was going to need a student loan and at the same time, I had realized that I probably would not be able to take on a full course load and it would take me several years to finish my degree. Luckily, my job was flexible enough to allow me to work part-time after I had given them notice that I would be attending school in the coming semester. With my disability, I had learned early on that things I wanted and needed would have to be planned well in advance for everything to get done before the deadlines. So, I had planned well before the semester to obtain my student loan.

The **Canada Student Loans Program** partners with the Canadian Government and most provinces and territories to help aide full- or part-time students that have low- or moderate-

> Student Loans –
> are loaned monetary funds that help students cover the cost of tuition, books, and living expenses. This type of loan usually has lower interest than other types and repayment on the loan is deferred while the student is educating.

income, dependents, or disabilities. A full course load for students with disabilities is 40% of a normal full course load. So if I took 2 classes per semester (out of the 5 that is considered to be a normal full course load) I would be considered a full-time student under their definition for students with disabilities. I was able to apply online and also check my loan application status online. At the same time that applied for the student loan, I was automatically assessed for student grants from the Government of Canada. In my application I had to also mail them certification that addressed my disability in order to obtain the most financial assistance that I can get by way of government grants. A *Letter of Assessment* was mailed out to let me know that I had qualified for the loan. Later on I also received a *Certificate of Eligibility* let me know how much I had qualified for. I submitted a signed copy of my *Certificate of Eligibility* as well as a void cheque so that I would be able to receive my loan deposits directly into my bank account.

The **Canada Access Grant for Students with Permanent Disabilities** was able to provide $2000 for me for the academic year for books and tuition. Up to $8000 per year was available for disabled students through another grant—the **Canada Study Grant for the Accommodation of Students with Permanent Disabilities**. This grant is able to provide services and equipment such as tutoring, technical aids, and special transportation. I was not eligible for the maximum on this grant, but I was still able to obtain some funds for equipment that would help me in school.

The student loan I obtained gave me a break due to my disability. I had close to 10 years to repay this special loan for students with disabilities. With the number of courses I had decided to take, it would take me at least 6 to 7 years to complete all the required courses to my degree. Even with that it was great to have at least 2 or 3 years to work full time and try to repay as much as I could out of the loan. If, in the future, I was unable to repay my loan I would register for a program called **Repayment Assistance Plan for Borrowers with Permanent Disabilities (RAP-PD)**. This program is able to help me by allowing me to pay back what I can reasonably afford. Depending on my family income and disability-incurred costs, each loan repayment would not exceed 20% of my income. In some cases, I may not have to make any loan repayment until my income increases.

Grants –
are monetary funds given to the student from the government, corporations, or foundations. Eligibility varies widely in requirements such as academic achievement, financial need, athletic skill, or special abilities. The student does not cessarily need to be undergoing education at the present time to receive this.

When I had finished the loan application process and found some free time between work hours, I had arranged to speak with an adviser at my former university. He told me about the **Ontario Student Assistance Program (OSAP)** website which gave me more options about the types of financial aide I might qualify for as a student and resident of Ontario. One program that was specific to my situation was the **Bursary for Students with Disabilities**. If eligible, this bursary would entitle me to $2000 per academic year for additional equipment or additional educational costs that may be incurred due to my disability. I was able to apply to this through my school's office with the

Bursaries –
are grants provided by the school to help pay for education-incurred fees. There are two types of bursaries: The first type is eligible to students whose parents' income is under a certain average threshold; a full bursary is given to students on the lowest end of this spectrum and partial bursaries are given up to the threshold. The second type of bursary is a monetary award given to students usually based on above average academic performance but can include other components as well – these are also known as scholarships.

appropriate documentation from my doctor. My adviser also told me about a website called DisabilityAwards.ca. When I got home and browsed through it, I realized there were tons of scholarships I was eligible for. I registered for their site so I could keep track of which ones I had applied for and I began browsing through them so I could get a head start on the applications, and also so I wouldn't miss the tight deadlines that some of them had.

I had a lot of help through the first years of my disability, a lot of which I didn't think I deserved because I hadn't come to terms with it yet. I'm glad I had so much support though, because looking back I knew I wouldn't have been able to do it all by myself. However, I learned a lot about myself those first few years. More than I had the last 10 years. I learned that if I was going to continue to enjoy my life, then I needed to take this disability seriously and if I wasn't going to, I shouldn't expect others to take me seriously. That was when I realized I wanted to become independent and start doing things for myself and that was also when I really started researching how I would be able to do what I wanted to. My biggest problem was finding the balance between being independent and being able to afford it. Many of the government programs that I unearthed was able to get me started and I was thankful for that. The Canadian government was able to get me back into a workplace that accommodated my disabilities and that really helped me overcome my financial situation. During this "process" (what I refer to as my first years with the disability) I learned that my earned income wasn't subject to tax due to how low my income was and the tax credit that I received from attending post-secondary would give me a tax break in my future years if my income were to increase. I was also lucky that I could keep my job part-time while attending school "full-time." As a disabled student, I didn't need to take on as heavy of a course load to be considered full-time. This enabled me to focus on my studies and, with time, pass all of my courses to complete my degree. My parents were extremely proud of me. I didn't even think that I would ever have a chance to finish my university degree, but as it turns out, I was able to accomplish many things by and for myself even with my handicap. I had a new view of my own self worth. With my new degree I was able to get a better paying position with much better benefits in the same company I was working for. It was great that they were able to offer me upwards mobility in spite of my disability and that I was able to change the opinion of many people in the company on what disabled people are capable of. Finishing school had been one of my last major goals. It took me 6 and a-half years to complete my degree and it gave me a new perspective to really appreciate hard work and dedication. With a new job and a degree to back it up, I had to look to a new adventure. I am continuing to learn more about finances to help me maintain my financial independence and I am also a huge advocate for students with disabilities. I spend my Thursday mornings at high schools with disabled and non-disabled perspective college students, telling them that it is never too late or too difficult to accomplish higher learning. I do this because I hope I can make an impact on that one student—a reflection of my past—to change his or her mind about being a disabled young adult.

Imagine being a normal student attending university or college full-time; it's a high-stress environment for the student to succeed and excel. Now imagine being stricken with a disability that you are faced to deal with for the rest of your life. As a disabled student your work load doubles, or even triples. You must go back and forth with physician visits, sort through paperwork so that you can continue receiving aid, work on homework assignments, study for exams, make deadlines, keep appointments. We understand that there is a great amount of frustration and anger that one must feel in the beginning of this situation. But after you've learned to heal from the grief you will no doubt have to start building your support network. Friends and family will help the healing process, but much of the work involved will still be up to you to accomplish. Dealing with the disability is a very time-consuming task. But you have the choice of learning to overcome your disabilities or be faced with the fact that one day they may overcome you. Remember that by choosing to take initiative in your struggles you are already halfway through the most difficult part of your disability. Whether you are a first-time student that is starting college or university, or you are continuing on the post-secondary path, we would like to congratulate you on your accomplishment. On the following pages we have outlined some of the federal aides that are available to disabled students and we hope with this small start we help you succeed in all your future endeavours.

☑   **Canada Student Loans for Students with Permanent Disabilities:** To Apply for the loan you must contact the National Student Loans Service Centre either by phone at **1-888-815-4514**, through their website, mail or through fax.

☑   **Canada Access Grant for Students with Permanent Disabilities:** To apply, you must first establish your financial need by applying and qualifying for a full-time or part-time Canada Student Loan. You must then complete and submit a separate application form for the Canada Study Grant for the Accommodation of Students with Permanent Disabilities. To find your province or territories Student Assistance office visit   http://www.canlearn.ca/eng/main/help/contact/cao. shtml or any educational institution to apply for loans and receive the application form for the Canada Study Grant.

☑   **Canada Study Grant for the Accommodation of Students with Permanent Disabilities:** This is another grant for students that must be applied through your province or territories Student Assistance office found at the link above.

☑   **Bursary for Students with Disabilities:**
You have two options to apply for this grant, you can either get the application from this website at https://osap.gov. on.ca/OSAPPortal/en/A-ZListofAid/UCONT004257.html or you can go to the staff at your university and speak with someone Office for Students with Disabilities and financial aid office for assistance.

☑ **Bursary for Students with Disabilities Attending Out-of-Country Postsecondary Institutions:**
The deadline to apply for this bursary is 30 days after class has started. To apply either call **1-807-343-7257**, email at tdd@osap.gov.on.ca or if you have difficulty with hearing you can contact **1-800-465-3958**.

☑ **Repayment Assistance Plan for Borrowers with Permanent Disabilities:** To apply contact the National Student Loans Service Centre (**1-888-815-4514**) to confirm your eligibility and you can either request the application while you speak with them or you may visit their website at https://nslsc.canlearn.ca/eng/default.aspx

☑ **Permanent Disability Benefit**: To apply you must contact the National Student Loans Service for eligibility and request an application by phone **1-888-815-4514**

Resources

Federal/National Programs:

Canadian Pension Plan (CPP):

The Canadian Pension Plan is a mandatory deduction, usually automatically taken off of your paycheque along with Employment Insurance (EI). Every Canadian citizen over the age of 18 that has been or is employed pays into the CPP. The employee pays half and the employer pays half of this amount, if you a self-employed, you pay the full portion. The only time you do not make contributions is if you are not working, receiving CPP Disability payments, or CPP Retirement payments. As you reach age 70, you stop making contributions even if you are still working.

The CPP Disability payout is made monthly for individuals who have contributed before, but have become disabled now and are unable to work at any job on a regular basis.
Eligibility follows the criteria outline below:

- you are under 65 years of age
- you have a severe and prolonged disability as defined by CPP legislation
- you have earned a specific minimum amount (this amount is adjusted annually)
- you have contributed to the CPP in four of the last six years at or above the minimum level of earnings, or three of the last six years if you have contributed at or above the minimum level of earnings for at least 25 years

If you do not meet the above criteria, it is less likely you will receive CPP payouts. Below are some exceptions that may allow you to receive CPP payouts if the following situations have applied to you:
- stayed at home and raised my children
- applied too late for a CPP disability benefit
- separated or divorced
- lived and worked in another country
- was physically or mentally unable to apply

It may take as long as 4 months to process your application. The benefit includes a fixed amount, plus an amount based on how much you contributed to the CPP during your entire working career. The maximum monthly payout for 2011 was $1,153.37 and the average payout was $810.46. Every January, there may be an increase in this amount to take into account an increase in the cost of living. The CPP Disability payout will be taxed as income.

For more information you can visit http://www.servicecanada. gc.ca/eng/isp/contact/contact_us.shtml
Or you may contact the Canadian Government toll free in Canada or the United States at: **1-800-277-9914**
TTY: **1-800-255-4786**

Canada Pension Plan Disability Vocational Rehabilitation Program

This program is designed to help people who receive the CPP Disability Benefit return to work by providing guidance and finding jobs, developing a return-to-work rehabilitation plan, and improving work skills or retraining for the work force. While this program is in effect, the CPP benefit holder is able to continue to receive benefits. If you are able to find a job, the CPP benefit will continue to be paid out for the first three months after work begins. If not, the benefit will stop at the end of the job search period.

For more information please call: **1-800-277-9914**
TTY: **1-800-255-4786** or visit http://www.servicecanada.gc.ca/eng/isp/pub/factsheets/vocrehab.shtml

Disability Tax Credit

This tax credit can apply as a deduction on individual's income tax if he or she is no longer a dependent. However, if the disabled individual is a dependent, the parent or guardian may use this as a deduction to his or her tax assessment by transferring the amount from the dependent.

Working Income Tax Benefit

This tax credit is applied as a deduction on your tax receipt if you are either over the age of 19 and you are a resident of Canada for the 2010 tax year and you made more than $3000.00 during the year. This is assuming that you have not attended a post secondary institution, and you do not have any dependants. If you have attended a post secondary institution and/or if you have a dependent such as a child you are still eligible to receive the tax credit.

Please visit http://www.cra-arc.gc.ca/bnfts/wtb/fq_qlfyng-eng.html#q1 for more details

Attendant Care Expense Deduction

The attendant care expense deduction is available to people who are entitled to claim the disability tax credit and who have paid for personal care that is necessary to enable them to work. People with a disability allowing them to receive the disability tax credit may also claim, under certain conditions, a deduction in computing net income for payments for attendant care enabling them to earn certain types of income. The maximum amount that may be claimed as a deduction is $5,000.

Home Buyers

The home buyers plan is sponsored by the Canadian government and it enables you to claim up to $5000.00 from the cost of the purchase of an eligible home. It is for people with disabilities only and it does not have to be the first time that you purchase a home. It is possible to get the credit if you are purchasing the home for a person who has disabilities

Residential Rehabilitation Assistance Program for Persons with Disabilities or (RRAP)

The RRAP can be applied for by Homeowners and landlords who qualify for assistance if the property is eligible. Your property may be eligible for RRAP-D if the property is currently occupied, or is going to be occupied by either a low income or person with disability. It is either rented or rents are less than the established levels for the area, is owned and the house is valued below a certain point, and finally meets minimum standards of health and safety.

Federal/National Scholarships/Bursaries for or related to Individuals with Disabilities:

Association of Universities & Colleges of Canada

The Association of Universities and Colleges is a gateway to various scholarships available throughout Canada. At the time of this book you are able to apply for over 150 scholarships through one website. For example they oversee the Mattinson Endowment Fund Scholarship for Disabled Students which can allow you to receive up to $2500 so long as you have been a resident of Canada for the last 2 years, have a permanent disability and keep at least a 75% average in your studies. They can be contacted either through their website of http://www.aucc.ca or through calling them at **(613) 563-1236**

DisabilityAwards.ca

"Lack of access to financial aid and lack of awareness of available financial aid opportunities are cited as the top two financially-related barriers to the completion of post-secondary education by students with disabilities."

This is an excellent website geared towards giving scholarships to Canadian students with disabilities. It allows you to search for disability-specific awards as well as specify your province of residency, province of study, and college intended to study at. This type of search will allow you to view awards that you are eligible for in your province of residency even though you intend to study in a different province. You can register on this website to save which awards you are interested in applying for and which awards you have already applied for. This website also gives detailed information about federal and provincial or territorial student loans, grants, or bursaries that are available to students with disabilities. Please visit http://disabilityawards.ca

If you would like more information about general post-secondary education in Canada you can visit http://www.studentawards. com/canlearn/

Repayment Assistance Plan for borrowers with a Permanent Disability (RAP-PD)

Students with permanent disabilities who are having difficulty paying back their student loans are eligible for this repayment plan. Under this program loan payments are based on family income, family size and disability related expenses, will not exceed 20% of their income, and in some cases will not need to be made until the student's income increases. Also, no student with a permanent disability will have a repayment period longer than 10 years.

For more information you can visit http://www.canlearn.ca/eng/after/repaymentassistance/rppd.shtml

You may also wish to contact the National Student Loans Service Centre
Within North America: **1-888-815-4514**
Outside North America: **1-800-2-225-2501**
TTY: **1-888-815-4556**

Permanent Disability Benefit

Students with severe permanent disabilities are eligible for the Permanent Disability Benefit. Borrowers must enrol by contacting the National Student Loans Service Centre, those that qualify for this loan may have their loans immediately forgiven.

The Canada Student Loans Program defines a severe permanent disability as "a functional limitation caused by a physical or mental impairment that prevents a borrower from performing the daily activities necessary to participate in studies at a post-secondary school level and the labour force and is expected to remain with the person for their expected life." Students with a severe permanent disability who received loans between 1995 and 2000 are eligible for immediate loan forgiveness regardless of when the severe permanent disability occurred, providing they meet the eligibility criteria and their loan remains with the financial institution. Borrowers who received student loans before 2000 can ask for an application from their financial institution and submit the completed application to their financial institution.

Note: Students in Ontario do not qualify for the Permanent Disability Benefit.

Please contact the National Student Loans Service Centre **1-888-815-4514** for information about your eligibility for this benefit. You may request an application by phone.

Provincial Programs:

Ontario Works

If you are in temporary financial need, Ontario Works can provide you with monthly income and help you find a job. This program is not only available for disabled or newly disabled individuals, but for all Ontario residents that cannot afford the basic necessities of life. Eligible individuals also receive prescription drug and dental coverage, eyeglasses, diabetic supplies, moving or eviction costs, employment-related costs (ex. transportation, child-care while working), and/or employment assistance to help you prepare for your job. To be eligible to receive help from Ontario Works, you must live in Ontario and need money right away to help pay for food and housing costs, and be willing to take part in activities that will help you find a job. The amount of money you may receive from Ontario Works will depend on your family size, income, assets, and housing costs. The Eligibility Estimator (http://appow.mcss.gov.on.ca/EligibilityEstimator/index.aspx) on the Ontario Works website can help you find out if you qualify for Ontario Works benefits. Depending on your outcome, you may have to contact your local Ontario Works office. Outlined below are some Ontario Works programs that may be pertinent to individuals with disabilities:

- Community Start Up and Maintenance Benefit: You should take advantage of this benefit if you are deciding to move to a new residence, if you are facing eviction fines, or if you are unable to pay rent, utility, or heating costs. You may be able to receive money from Ontario Works to help with these costs but the amount you receive will depend on the size of your family.

•Guide Dogs: For individuals that own a certified guide dog, Ontario Works may be able to pay for the dog's care.

•Special Services at Home: This program helps families who are caring for a child with a developmental or physical disability, as well as adults with a developmental disability. It will help your family pay for special services in your home or outside of your home as long as your child is not receiving support from a residential program. For example, you can hire someone to help your child learn new skills and abilities, such as improving their communications skills to do more of the daily living activities on their own. Families can also get help to pay for services that will give them a break from the day-to-day care of their child. The amount you receive depends on the type and amount of service your child needs, what help is available in the community, and what kind of support your family is already receiving.

Assistance for Children with Disabilities:

If you are a parent caring for a child with a severe disability, you may be able to receive some financial help. The Assistance for Children with Severe Disabilities Program helps parents with some of the extra costs of caring for a child who has a severe disability. If you are a parent of legal guardian whose child is younger than 18 years old, lives at your home, and has a severe disability, you may be eligible to receive help under this program depending on your income. Parents can get between $25 and $440 a month to help with costs, such as travel to doctors and hospitals, special shoes and clothes, parental relief, wheelchair repairs, assistive devices, hearing aids, hearing aid batteries, prescription drugs, dental care, eyeglasses. How much you are eligible for depends on your family's income, severity of the disability, the kind of difficulties your child has when walking, communicating, feeding himself or bathing himself and the extraordinary costs related to the disability.

Opportunities Fund for Persons with Disabilities

A funding contribution is provided to individuals, employers and organizations, to help people with disabilities prepare for, obtain and maintain employment or self-employment. It is meant for individuals who are unable to receive Employment Insurance (EI) and it helps overcome the barriers that one may face in the market for jobs. For example the opportunities fund can help you start your own business, increase your job skills, help you integrate into the workplace through services that meet your special needs, and through encouraging employers to provide you with work opportunities and experience to better your life. This fund offers three funding categories for projects involving eligible activities: Financial Assistance for Individuals, Funding for Employers and Organizations for Local and Regional Projects and Funding for Organizations for National Projects.

For more information on Ontario Works and a list of phone numbers by municipality, please visit http://www.mcss.gov. on.ca/en/mcss/programs/social/ow/index.aspx

For more information about Ontario's Disability Support Program and a list of phone numbers by municipality, please visit http://www.mcss.gov.on.ca/en/mcss/programs/social/odsp/ index.aspx

Co-Op and Non-Profit Housing

To find the community housing groups in your area visit the website http://www.onpha.on.ca/AM/Template. cfm?Section=Access_Centres. The community housing is meant to allow seniors to continue living in their own communities and enables people living on low income a place to live. This includes those who are disabled seeking independence and those people who have difficulty finding an affordable place to live.

Provincial Scholarships and Bursaries:

Dr. Albert Rose Bursary:

This bursary helps Ontario's social housing tenants with the cost of post-secondary. This bursary is eligible to Ontario residents in two award types: The Full Bursary, which pays a maximum one-time sum of $3,000, and the Part Bursary, which pays a maximum of $1,000. The awarded amount is based on the number of qualified applicants, meaning more than one individual may receive the bursary in the given year. Eligibility for the Full Bursary are limited to students entering their first or second year of a post-secondary institution full-time leading to a degree, certificate, or diploma. The Part Bursary applies to those enrolled in trades or skills program that is at least 4 weeks in length, those enrolled in an adult learning program, or first or second year part-time students enrolled in a post-secondary program. Students who have received the Dr. Albert Rose Bursary are not eligible to apply again.

For more information, further instructions, and an online application form, please visit: http://www.mah.gov.on.ca/Page6371.aspx To contact them directly, E-mail bursary.mah@ontario.ca or call **(416) 585-6021**

Justin Eves Foundation Scholarship

The primary goal of the Justin Eves Foundation to assist post secondary students with their education through scholarships. Students may apply for assistance for up to two years of their course of study, and are eligible to receive up to $3000 per year. The scholarship is only available to those students who went to a secondary school in Ontario.

To apply for the scholarship go to the following link and complete the application at http://www.justinevesfoundation.com

you
or your
spouse
becomes disabled

Chapter 4

Chapter 4
You or Your Spouse becomes Disabled

We had never thought this would happen to us, especially since we were so young and worry-free. Suddenly, a whole burden of issues was upon us. Our dreams were shattered and our lives came to a standstill, but what was most trying of all was the financial strain it brought to our relationship.

Last year on our way to our favourite winter getaway we were involved in a head-on collision which immobilized my wife, leaving her paralyzed from the waist down. I could not believe this was happening to us. We had only been married for a couple of years. Her parents lived outside of the country and could offer almost no help, let alone financial support for our exponentially increasing medical bills. My own mother was on a limited pension and could do little else but to take care of her daughter-in-law when I was called back to work. Our entire savings for a new home had been depleted within months of going to therapies that were greatly needed, but uninsured by health care, and we were getting more and more desperate in finding ways to manage with this draining new lifestyle.

"It was draining. Every moment of it was draining. It was physically draining, it was mentally draining. I can only imagine what it might have been like for her."

Our relationship almost fell apart. We felt frustrated with each other. As much as I wanted, I felt like I couldn't be there for her when she needed and she was constantly angry at herself for putting us in a financial sinkhole. However, that was just an excuse for what she really felt. Deep down she was frightened and distraught that she had permanently lost the ability to stand, walk, run, and many other things she used to enjoy.

To our relief, her parents had flown overseas to be with her as soon as they learned of the accident and I think that their presence and teamwork really helped us hold it together.

The disability really took a toll on our finances. Most of our savings, earnings, and insurance payouts were put towards her physical recovery so we had little left for private counselling. My wife's family doctor was able to find a psychiatrist that was covered under our provincial health care to help her with depression. When my work performance started to decline, I knew I had to take some time off and get help. My boss was very understanding as he had been through a similar situation with his stroke-ridden mother. He had granted me time off work and pointed me to some useful resources, including my company's employee support and distress line.

Being the primary caregiver during these difficult times, I found it very challenging to stay positive for my wife. But she needed just that, especially in the beginning. If I couldn't be there for her to vent out her frustrations and shed her tears then I wasn't doing my job and we would never be able to pull through this together.

At first, it was the emotional aspect of the disability. It was the anger, grief, frustration and the exhaustion of it all. Our individual counselling helped us learn how to cope with ourselves, but our couples counselling really made an impact about each other.

While we were healing emotionally, we began to accept the disability as a part of our lives. It was not her disability to deal with alone, it was our disability because I am just as involved in it as she is. We now see it as just another chapter in life and we know that there are many others like us, so we look to them for inspiration and knowledge.

Once we began our new outlook on life, we had enough peace-of-mind to start tackling our diminishing finances. The thing that made a major difference in our disability was that we were assigned to an amazing social worker. She made many months worth of research on financial programs into a well introduced step-by-step process that only took a few weeks to understand and a couple more to get started. What she started with was the **Disability Tax Credit**, the **Canadian Pension Plan Disability Benefits**, and **Employment Insurance**. These programs are the backbone of disability-related support offered by the government. In particular, individuals that are eligible for the Disability Tax Credit will have an easier time applying for other types of government-funded support programs. By starting the application for these programs she had helped us an astronomical amount to get the ball rolling. Once we acquired the tools and knowledge and gained the motivation, we went with the momentum and took it one step further to ensure our financial future.

My wife was working as an airline stewardess before the accident. She was enrolled in her company's insurance plan and was supposed to receive her long-term disability pay outs on a bi-monthly basis. However, much to our dismay, we discovered that her company had a very select plan that would only cover her for 2 years under what they called "regular occupation" which, as we had explained to us, meant that she cannot perform her regular job duties. After the 2 year period was over we were told she would not be eligible for coverage as the plan switched to "any occupation" definition, which meant if she could do any form of work she would be denied coverage. Because we had never thought an accident like this would happen we did not apply for a supplementary plan. A supplementary plan would have allowed us to get coverage after her 2 year period had expired. Since we were the ones paying the insurance premium out-of-pocket we would not have a tax hit on what she got back from the insurance company. If her employer had paid for the premiums, we would have had to pay taxes on the insurance money received after the accident.

When my wife left her job, we made sure that her vacation pay and bonuses were paid out to us. Every little bit counted and we needed to make sure it was accounted for. However, even this small amount of income was not enough to support her new lifestyle. We knew there was financial aid out there so the obvious next step was to start looking.

As residents of British Columbia for most of our life we were required to enrol in the **Medical Services Plan (MSP)**. This provincial program covers many prescription drugs (via Fair PharmaCare), hospital benefits, and subsidized fees or discounts for ambulance services and medical aide while travelling. Both my wife and I pay premiums into this mandatory plan, which are thus deducted on our paycheques. My wife's supplemental group insurance through her company usually covered additional prescription costs.

After becoming disabled, we applied for **Persons with Disabilities Assistance**—a financial program provided by the government of British Columbia. Approval for this program gave us a maximum of approximately $700 per month. In addition, my wife received a no-deductible coverage for Fair PharmaCare and coverage of other medical services such as optical and dental.

We found that the **Aids to Independent Living** program through the Canadian Red Cross was able to supply medical equipment for loan to eligible individuals. Her physiotherapist was able to refer her to this program and based on her low income, she was able to qualify for this program. There were new and used equipment for loan and the loan period is for as long as a person needs it. The list of equipment for loan is quite extensive and we were able to get a wheelchair, bed assists, and bath and toilet aids, as well as grab rails.

We applied for the **Canadian Pension Plan Disability Benefits** which gave us a monthly payout from her CPP contributions over the years that she had been employed. We had thought to apply for **Employment Insurance (EI)** as well but after looking into it, we found out that the amount of money that she was able to receive from her insurance company would be taken into effect. Since the insurance company payout was pretty high, she wouldn't be able to receive any of her EI contributions. Unfortunately, in the case of EI, eligibility requires you to have worked 600 hours in the last 52 weeks to be considered for this payout. Since my wife's insurance company would be paying for 104 weeks, we would not be eligible for EI during her disability.

During my search of government programs and financial assistance, I came upon the **Canadian Mortgage and Housing Corporation (CMHC)**. I knew about this organization before, when my wife and I were thinking about purchasing our own home, but I had no idea they would be able to help with our disability, especially since we were renting. Luckily, our landlord is also my parents-in-law, who legally owned the home under their name, but let us live in it by taking care of the property and paying very little for rent. Seeing first-hand the difficulty of their daughter's situation, they had insisted that rent was to be put to a halt until we could get back on our feet again. Although they were semi-retired and separated by distance, my parents-in-law offered whatever assistance they could. When I broke the good news that assistance for home modifications could be obtained, they were elated and very eager to immediately begin modifications to their home for my wife's sake. They trusted whatever modifications needed to us to decide. It didn't matter to them what we did with the home, as long as my wife would have an easier time performing day-to-day tasks.

Following my in-laws' approval, I applied for the **Residential Rehabilitation Assistance Program for Persons with Disabilities (RRAP-D)** on their behalf. Because my wife's parents were the landlords of the property, they would be able to receive up to a maximum of $24,000 in loan for modifications to the house to assist my wife with her with mobility. These would include ramps to get into the home as well as height adjustments for countertops and hand rails.

Our next step was to speak to a financial adviser in our community. What other sorts of financial support can we find? Is there hidden income where we hadn't thought of looking? The **Registered Disability Savings Plan (RDSP)** was like an investment account which earned tax-free interest with the added benefit of income support from the federal government. Much to my surprise the plan gives up to $1000.00 yearly just for having the account open. The first contribution of up to $500 maximum from my own pocket will be matched by the federal government in a 3-to-1 fashion (the government would contribute $1500), the next contribution of up to $1000 maximum is matched 2-to-1 (a potential government contribution of $2000). I was told that if we needed the money in the future, we would be able to withdraw it tax-free. There are restrictions though. One of the restrictions is that generally, the funds contributed by the government must remain the account for a minimum of 10 years before they can be withdrawn, however certain exceptions apply.

Another restriction deals with the type of investments we hold. An investment such as the Guaranteed Investment Certificate (GIC) cannot be withdrawn before the maturity date, which is a pre-determined future date at the time of purchase. To take full advantage of this program it would have been wiser to open the account sooner to have collected the interest, but since registering for the account, I have been making monthly contributions towards this plan on my wife's behalf. We are planning for the future and given this great opportunity, we want to be ready for it.

As the end of the tax year approached, my wife started to look into tax deductions and credits that could be claimed on behalf of her disability and expenses. My wife was already enrolled for the **Disability Tax Credit**, but I was able to claim this tax deduction as her spouse to reduce my taxable income since I was the sole income-earner now. In addition to this claim, I was also able to file what is called a **Spouse or Common-law Partner Amount**. I am able to claim this amount because my wife's net income of the year was under $10,000. The **Medical Expense Tax Credit** was also claimed under my income tax. This claim was filed because the bathroom aides, along with dental and optical examinations, prescribed physiotherapy, premiums on our health insurance plans, and ineligible prescription drugs were paid for out-of-pocket by my wife and me. Again, I was able to transfer this amount onto my taxes.

In late spring, almost six months after my wife's injury, she told me that she had been looking into finding new employment opportunities for herself. I wasn't surprised because I knew she was the type that couldn't stand being at home, unable to do anything. Before the accident, she had been a very active person and very independent as well. I knew it was time for her to move on, but I didn't expect it to be so soon.

My mother had already left two months prior as my wife had re-learned how to do all the daily tasks very quickly; she was even cooking simple meals for us. I have to give my wife credit, because she had found most of the information, in terms of financial aid, about her disability. She had also filed our taxes for us because she felt it was "the least that she could do" being a home keeper. Her desire to get out of the house and, once again, become an income-earner, was strong, so she had started looking on the internet for resources to employ people with disabilities.

What she discovered was that the Canadian Government offered a program for people with disabilities who are currently receiving CPP payments. The program is called the **Disability Vocational Rehabilitation Program** and it would allow my wife to get training for a different job while being paid. Unfortunately her disability would not allow her to go back to her old profession. But with this program she was able to get training to work in the call centre of her former employer and they were happy to welcome her back. Because my wife already had the background and knowledge about the company, her training took half of the time required. She was able to get back to work in a couple of weeks and this meant a lot to her.

She discovered that she would be able to get a yearly bus pass for $45 that was specifically subsidized by the B.C. government for disabled individuals. This allowed her to go to work and attain a greater sense of independence as she would not have to rely on me for her transportation. Another program that we looked at offered a $500 rebate off the provincial tax on gasoline if we were driving, however we weighed the costs and since we had access to transit we decided to go with the latter. In the long run it would prove to be a wiser financially, especially since the cost of purchasing another vehicle for my wife would be more than we could afford.

During this whole experience of trying to find a balance between taking our life back, securing our finances for the future, and many, many painstaking hours spent organizing the paperwork, we were able to come out of it with more knowledge and in much better shape than if we had given up. Neither my wife, nor I, nor any of our close relatives knew that there would be so many helping hands out there for people with disabilities.

We are slowly starting to feel more financially stable, but evermore confident in our abilities to play the cards that were dealt to us. What I mean is that coming out of this, we have learned more about finances than we would ever have thought possible. We discovered our potential as a couple as well as our innate ability to strive on bettering ourselves and overcoming whatever obstacles we are faced with. We are once again beginning to build our dream again. We want to be homeowners one day and we want to have a family.

The amount of money that we were able to save was phenomenal. The amount of support that we had was more than we could ever ask for. In the next few months we will be acquiring our first home together, and soon after, having our first child. Even though my wife is disabled, she is still very able to be a wonderful, loving mother to our baby. We will continue to wisely invest our money and seek out ways to have fun while on a tight budget. For the first time in many months, I feel confident that we will be okay.

☑ Disability Tax Credit: To apply, fill out Form T2201, Disability tax credit certificate and return it to the Canadian Revenue Agency.

☑ Canadian Pension Plan Disability Benefits: The application for disability benefits is available on the CRA website or you can call and request the application package be mailed to you through either service in English: **1-800-277-9914** or service in French: **1-800-277-9915**

☑ Employment Insurance: To apply for EI benefits you may either visit the service Canada website or visit a service Canada Centre near you to gain assistance with the application. You will need your SIN, former employers address and other information that will assist you in your application.

☑ Residential Rehabilitation Program for Persons with Disabilities: To apply to this program either visit the CMHC website at http://www.cmhc-schl.gc.ca/en/co/prfinas/prfinas_016.cfm or call CMHC at **1-800-668-2642**

☑ Registered Disability Savings Plan: You must be eligible to receive the disability tax credit, be under 60 years of age, have a SIN number and be a Canadian Resident, then all you are required to do is to contact your local financial institution to open an account.

☑ Disability Vocational Rehabilitation Program: If you are already receiving the Canadian Pension Plan Disability Benefit all you need to do to apply for this is call **1-800-277-9914**

Disability Tax Credit

This tax credit reduces the income tax that a person with a disability has to pay. It is a good idea to transfer a portion or the entire claim to your spouse, common-law partner, or another person that supports your living expenses if you have low or no income. The person with the disability must apply for this credit by having a qualified practitioner, such as a family doctor, fill out part of the Tax Credit Certificate.

Spouse or Common-law Partner Amount

A tax deduction can be made if you supported your spouse or common-law partner and his or her net income was less than $10,382. This federal tax amount that you're eligible to receive can be calculated on line 303. Remember to also claim the corresponding provincial or territorial tax credit. Only either you or your spouse or common-law partner may claim this amount. Both of you cannot claim this amount for each other for the same tax year.

For more information, you can visit the Canada Revenue Agency website at http://www.cra-arc.gc.ca/ or call **1-800-959-8281**

Medical Expense Tax Credit

A tax credit that can be claimed for you, your spouse or common-law partner, or your or your spouse's dependent children born in 1993 or later. Eligible medical expenses incurred by any of the above individuals may be claimed on your federal tax return on line 330. If you are claiming for a dependent not listed above, complete the claim on line 331. For a list of eligible medical expenses, please visit the Canada Revenue Agency website.

Canadian Pension Plan Disability Benefits

The Canada Pension Plan (CPP) disability benefit is available to people who have made enough contributions to the CPP, and whose disability prevents them from working at any job on a regular basis. The only way to receive the Canadian Pension Plan Disability Benefits is to apply in writing to service Canada. It can take up to four months before you hear if you have been granted the disability benefits.

Employment Insurance

This type of payout is eligible for a variety of people. If you are claiming maternity, parental, or sickness benefits, your eligibility includes that your regular weekly earnings have been decreased by more than 40% and that you have worked and paid into EI for 600 hours of the last 52 weeks or since your last claim. In certain situations, the qualifying period may be extended up to 104 weeks. Self-employed persons may also be eligible to receive EI for the above benefits.

As mentioned above, if you are receiving additional sources of income such as wage or salary commissions, bonuses, vacation or severance pay, retirement pension, insurance coverage, self-employment income, or investment income, you may not be entitled to receive Employment Insurance or the amount that your receive will be less.

Compassionate care benefits are eligible to individuals that are temporarily away from work in order to provide care or support to a family member who is gravely ill or with a significant risk of death. When this benefit is combined with maternity, parental, or sickness benefits, the individual may be eligible to receive up to a maximum of 71 weeks.

The basic benefit rate is 55% of your average earnings up to a yearly maximum of $44,200 paid out to you. You will receive EI payouts bi-weekly but you must report to the program every two weeks to inform them of any earned income. The maximum payment is $468 per week. Higher benefit rates are given to low-income families with children that have an income of less than $25,921. Be aware that the insurance amount paid is taxable and the taxes will automatically be deducted from your payment. You may apply for Canadian Pension Plan Disability Benefits together with Employment Insurance.

For more detailed information about Employment Insurance, dial **1-800-206-7218** or please visit: http://www.servicecanada.gc.ca/eng/sc/ei/index.shtml

Canadian Mortgage and Housing Corporation (CMHC)

This Canadian corporation is a provider of mortgage loan insurance, mortgage-backed securities, housing policies and programs, and housing research. They help enhance Canada's housing finance options and also assist Canadians who cannot afford housing in the private market. Any future or current homeowner should access this site for more information about buying a home, mortgage insurance, as well as renting, maintaining, or renovating a home. They also offer several programs for financial assistance regarding your home or rental property.

Visit their website for more information: http://www.cmhc-schl.gc.ca/en/index.cfm

Residential Rehabilitation Program for Persons with Disabilities

This is one of the programs offered by the CMHC. This type of financial assistance offers homeowners and landlords a fully forgivable loan to pay for modifications to may their property more accessible to persons with disabilities. Examples of eligible modifications include ramps, handrails, chair lifts, bath lifts, height adjustment for countertops, and cues for doorbells or fire alarms. The loan amount will vary according to the geographic zone and whether you are a homeowner or a landlord. Additionally, you may also apply for financial assistance to address structural and system repairs to the property.

For additional information and how to apply visit: http://www.cmhc-schl.gc.ca/en/co/prfinas/prfinas_003.cfm
or call **1-800-668-2642**

Disability Vocational Rehabilitation Program

This program is designed to help you get back to work if you are receiving the Canadian Disability Pension benefits by granting you providing you with guidance through access to a Vocational Specialist. This specialist will work with you to develop a return to work program and to help you improve your skills and retrain. The specialist will also help you develop your resume, assist you with your job search and get you on the right track to working again.

Fair PharmaCare

Is a program that the provincial government of British Columbia has developed to ensure that all residents of British Columbia who qualify will be able to receive the drugs they need. It covers many prescription drugs and some medical supplies but it does set a maximum on what it will cover, and just how much of each prescription or medical supplies will be covered varies. PharmaCare sets a maximum cost that it will recognize for eligible prescription drugs and dispensing fee and medical supplies. There is a family deductible based on household income. Which means that if your family earns more than $15,000 you will have to pay the entire cost of the drugs up front until you reach the deductible limit which will entitle you to a 70% cost reduction on drugs.

Persons with Disabilities Assistance

This program is designed to assist those disabled who are unable to return to the work force and provides income assistance to give you security of income and increased participation within the community. You are able to receive between $531 to $1043.06 per month depending on your circumstances and depending on your living circumstances. To apply to receive the benefit you must fill out the Persons with Disabilities Designation application and send to the Ministry of Social Development, Health Assistance Branch.

BC Family Bonus (BCFB)

The BCFB program includes the basic family bonus and the BC Earned Income Benefit. This program provides non-taxable amounts paid monthly to help low- and modest-income families with the cost of raising children under 18 years of age. Benefits are combined with the CCTB into a single monthly payment.

Aids to Independent Living

To be eligible for the Aids to independent living you must be referred to occupational therapist, homecare nurse, physiotherapist, or other health unit staff. You must also undergo a financial eligibility test to ensure that you require the assistance, and are not gaming the system. The eligibility test indicates that you need to have less than $20,000 in savings and make less than $20,000 a year. Equipment is not available if you live in an extended care facility such as a nursing home. Applications are made on your behalf by medical staff.

Basic Family Bonus

The basic family bonus is calculated based on the number of children you have and your adjusted family net income. Use the child and family benefits online calculator which can be found at http://www.cra-arc.gc.ca/benefits-calculator/ to determine the amount of you are able to receive.

BC Earned Income Benefit

Families whose working income is more than $10,000 and whose adjusted family net income is $21,480 or less, may also be entitled to the following amounts:
- $8.41 per month for the first child;
- $7.08 per month for the second child; and
- $12.00 per month for each additional child.

Families whose working income is between $3,750 and $10,000 or whose adjusted family net income is more than $21,480 may get part of the earned income benefit. You may use the Child and family benefits calculator to determine the benefits that you are able to receive. This program is fully paid for by the Province of British Columbia and if you wish for more information call **1-800-387-1193**

Housing Matters BC –

Through Housing Matters BC an individual who is living on low income (which often times is someone who has a disability) will be able to apply to the Rental Assistance Program which provides direct cash assistance to assist with the cost of renting. The average payment per family is around $350 per month but it can range anywhere between $50 up to a maximum of $875 per month. You are only eligible to receive the assistance if you are working and are making less than $35,000

Trusts –

Within British Columbia it is possible to have a high net worth and still receive disability assistance, despite going above the asset threshold for credits; this would be called using a Trust. A trust is a legal relationship where someone (the trustee) holds the legal interest in (legally owns) money or other assets for someone else's benefit (that person is called the "beneficiary"). The legal relationship is often, but not always, described in a written agreement, or in a will. There can be more than one trustee, and multiple beneficiaries, or there may be only one of each. For instance you may hire someone to look after your assets as a trustee, the trustee will act in the best interest of the beneficiary which does not have to be you, it may be your child, spouse or even your parents if you so choose.

Please keep in mind that your employment and assistance worker is not a lawyer. He or she cannot advise you how or whether to put funds in a trust. You should obtain independent legal advice if you wish to create a trust, or if you seek information about trusts that is specific to your situation. There are two basic forms of trusts a discretionary trust indicates that you have no direct control over the assets in the account, the trustee makes all the decisions for you, and works in your best interest. They also choose when to pay out assets and what to invest in. It is possible that if you begin a trust using over $100,000 of your own money (and if you are the beneficiary) it will still be counted as an asset for the purposes of receiving disability assistance. A Non Discretionary trust gives the beneficiary some more control, however as you continue to have control over the assets it will limit the benefit of using the trust for the purpose of receiving disability assistance.

Income assistance –

Residents of B.C. who are disabled may be eligible to receive income assistance in two different forms. You may be eligible to receive "shelter" rates, which is to say you may be eligible to receive help for either renting or owning your own home. The range that you may receive depending on eligibility and the type of home is from $375.00 to $820. You may also be eligible to receive income assistance if you meet the qualifications. The self serve assessment is a simple web tool that should inform you on whether you are eligible to receive the income assistance or not. To take the self serve assessment, go to the following website http://www.hsd.gov.bc.ca/bcea.htm. Or you may use the below phone numbers for assistance over the phone.

For Income Assistance information and services please call toll free **1-866-866-0800** or visit your local Employment and Income Assistance Office.

your
parents
are disabled

Chapter 5

Chapter 5
Your Parents Are Disabled

Right around my 47th birthday I started to notice that my parents were having greater difficulty with their daily tasks, especially my father who appeared to be suffering from what he called "momentary memory lapses". I was worried about his health but when I asked him he laughed it off, reminding me how his mind just likes to wander and that he was fine. I wasn't entirely satisfied with his answer so I asked my mother if there was anything going on with Dad that she needed help on, she said that everything was great and that it was sweet of me to worry.

I thought nothing of it for a few months until my mother, now well into her 80's, fell and broke her hip. I went to the hospital every day and my father was always with me, which, to me, was normal, since Dad was never away from Mom for any length of time. They had always been close, even when I was a child; their relationship set the standard of what I imagined mine to be like growing up. After each visit, I drove my father home and walked him back to the house. I didn't want to risk both of them getting hurt. He was always happy to have me there but always said goodbye at the door saying he was tired and needed to get to sleep. It wasn't until we brought my mother back home from the hospital that I knew there was something wrong with him.

Mom had been trying to hint that I didn't need to come in the house and that they would be fine, but I insisted on helping them out. When I entered, the house was an absolute mess and my mother broke down crying. I guess she had been taking care of my father since he was not quite there anymore when he was by himself. She said that he seemed to have better days whenever we would get together but she was too scared to talk to me about it. I was shocked, I knew my mother only wanted to protect my father but I think she did more damage than good. I wanted to take him to the doctor to get checked out so we would get a better idea of what was troubling him. My mother was more fearful than optimistic. She agreed only after a lot of persuading and pointing out that it would be best for both of them.

When we were able to get in to see their family doctor, he told us my father was suffering from dementia and likely had Alzheimer's disease. A CT scan would follow just to confirm the results. My mother was devastated by the news. She felt like she wouldn't be able to continue to take care of him at their current home, especially with all of the daily chores starting to pile up. She thought she would have to move, especially after her injury, because she no longer had the same mobility and could not rely on her husband for support.

Québec health insurance covers some medical services. One of their programs, **Devices That Compensate for Physical Deficiencies**, could help pay for the tools that she would require for mobility. The program would cover the costs of a wheel chair and canes, but not the cost of a motorized, or powered wheel chair. However, the program does cover the cost of the repair for such units, which made my mother more at ease about the purchase of an electronic wheel chair when the time came since she would not have to foot the entire bill for repairs. My mother liked the idea, but she wanted to put it off for a few months since she was still able to walk with a cane that she had purchased at her local drug store.

"I hoped that she wouldn't become stubborn if her mobility ever declined. I hoped that she would address her mobility issues without having another accident be the reason to address it."

For the time being, I began looking into ways that would help my parents be able to continue staying at home, but with additional aids to make their day-to-day tasks easier. There is a health information line in Québec. It is free and available 24 hours a day and 7 days a week, the phone number to dial is **8-1-1** and from there you will be connected to a health professional. My question was, is there any way for my parents, with their current conditions, to continue living at home by themselves? The nurse on the line told me that Québec health care has several support programs for the elderly that fall under the disabled definition. I discovered that if my parents were to stay in their home and make physical adjustments to their living condition, they would be eligible for a reimbursement for some of the costs involved in renovating their home to be more adaptive to their disabilities. The program is administered under Canadian Mortgage and Housing Corporation for people with disabilities. With their age, my parents also fall under another category: seniors 65 years or over that have difficulty with daily living activities. I looked into the financial support offered by this program and discovered that due to the way my parents' home was set up it would be more costly for them to change their home than to move into what I am told is a **<u>universal design</u>** living home. The universal design home is one in which there are no stairs or other obstacles, the home is easily accessible to people with reduced mobility, and everything is located on the ground level. This would enable my mother to, at least, have some freedom of movement, but there was still the issue of my father. I didn't know what we would be able to do for him. He was having problems remembering to turn

> "Universal design refers to broad-spectrum ideas meant to produce buildings, products and environments that are inherently accessible to both people without disabilities and people with disabilities." -*Wikipedia*

off the stove, the lights, and the tap and he was often forgetting where he left objects or what he had been doing moments ago. The drugs he was given were only preventing him from getting worse, not improving his condition. Thus, my mother had taken on his burden as well as her own. I knew my mother would need some help during the day so I looked into different programs that would get them in home care at reduced cost.

I discovered that Québec, our province of residence, offers a program that would reduce the cost of having a **caretaker** to come in and do some of the chores and work that my mother and dad used to do. The program is called **Financial Assistance for Domestic Help Services**, and it offers a base-value of $4 per hour of service regardless of income and then an additional $0.42 to $7 (a variable amount) depending on the level of income that my parents receive; in this case, their pension. The cost for this service varies depending on the qualifications of the person providing the service and what they are expected to do while maintaining the home. It is possible that if you hire a nurse, the cost will be higher than if you had hired someone whose training is not quite as extensive. The cost for a caretaker can range from under $20 to well over $40 an hour and they can be hired

People that are over 65 are automatically eligible to receive basic financial assistance for domestic help services of up to $4 per hour. The variable amount will depend on your income.

Income-splitting is useful when one spouse earns a larger income than the other and subsequently, would pay higher income tax. When you income-split, the taxes of the higher income earner can be reduced. One way to do this is for the higher income earner to contribute to a spousal registered retirement savings plan (SPRRSP). By contributing to any type of RRSP, one can have their income tax reduced. During retirement, these funds can be accessed, and in this particular case, the spouse will have retirement savings, even though he or she may not have earned income or personally contributed to the RRSP.

through health companies. Some of the caretakers can be responsible for doing all of the shopping and housework or even just sitting and spending time with the clients. This program would greatly help my parents and also, cause me to worry less about my mother leaving the house without my father. Since my father had a healthy pension, and my parents had undergone income splitting, they were not eligible for the full coverage. But my mother agreed that this sounded like an excellent program and we began the application process.

During the next couple of years, my parents' health continued on the decline. Both of my parents' hearing had decreased considerably, but they were unable to apply for hearing device coverage since their hearing had not degraded to the point where they could not function in society. My mother, being the stubborn woman that she could be, decided that she would pay for them out of her own pocket. The set that she ended up buying for my father was $3000 per ear. I was shocked that not only had she decided not to tell me she was going to buy them, but that she had spent so much on what would likely be lost by my poor dad. I do understand that, sometimes, you must spend a significant amount in order to get a quality set of hearing assistance devices and in this case my father did need to hear, especially since it was getting more and more difficult to talk with him because of his dementia. Nonetheless, I would have preferred for my parents to spend the money on something nice for themselves, like a little vacation. But I guess at their age with the current ongoing circumstances, they may as well have purchased an umbrella during a flood.

While looking for anything else that my mother may have tried to hide from me, I discovered that, for the last couple of months, she had been sending out a cheque for $300 to a so-called African prince. The return correspondence from him told her that he would be sending her a large sum of cash once he received processing funds from her. This was an obvious scam and I couldn't believe that my poor mother had fallen for it. This scam is just one of the many that target the elderly and mentally disabled. They always make an offer of a large sum of cash but before this amount can be received lawyer or legal fees, or some other type of funds have to be paid. Of course, the large return-payment is never made to you and you will not be able to contact them again once they have taken your money. During the whole process, though, they will not cease their communication with you and will persist in trying to get your money. When faced with one of these scams, the best way is to ignore them. There are variations to this scam, and the scammers are always trying to come up with new ways to swindle you out of your hard earned money. So if you receive emails, letters, or phone calls from organizations such as these always do a short internet search to discover their legitimacy. As well if it turns out they are scammers, there is a website dedicated to busting them and teaching them a lesson. Of course I discover all of this after my mother has sent these people several thousand dollars. There is often no way that you can get anything back from scammers and I had read several stories of people losing everything that they have to scam artists with no recourse available.

In order to try to help and protect my parents I asked them if I would be able to help look after their finances. It is not as easy as it seems. You'd think that all it involved was monitoring their bank accounts and spending, but I wanted to do more than that. I needed to monitor and restrict access when needed. This involved getting a legal power of attorney over their affairs and there was a very large shift in responsibility from them to me. It was very much like how when I was a child and my parents were trying to teach me the value of wealth. Only now, my parents were not bright-eyed youngsters but had lived very full lives without having had to worry about people taking advantage of them. I asked my mother specifically to check with me before making any donations. This, of course, did not make her happy since she thought I had lost my faith in her. I also knew that she felt like I was taking away her independence. But, that wasn't the case. I just knew that my parents were more trusting of people than they should have been and I didn't want her sending her hard earned pension to a fraudulent cause. Regardless, I now had power of attorney over their finances so I was able to prevent a few more cases of fraud that my parents would have fallen prey to.

In the next couple of months, I noticed that despite all of the medication, both prescription and supplement, both of my parents' health continued to deteriorate substantially. It got to be well past the point where I would be able to assist them in staying in their home, and a private nurse was becoming far more expensive than either my parents or I could afford. I began searching for a home where my parents would be able to be looked after 24/7. I looked at various living arrangements and attempted to find the one that would look after them and treat them with dignity. I knew that as unfortunate as it were, there are some places that did not treat their residents with the respect that they deserve, so I needed to make sure I could trust the home with my parents' twilight years.

"The problem wasn't finding a place for my parents to 'retire' into. The problem was changing my parents' mindset about these retirement homes. My mother was opposed to the idea; I knew where she was coming from though. She didn't want to lose her independence and her home that she had lived in for the past 40 years."

There were plenty of retirement homes. Many with reasonable monthly rental rates but some were less affordable than others. The elderly with lower pensions and income also had assistance from the government in what is known to be a subsidized retirement homes. Not all retirement homes were subsidized, only certain ones were. Because of my parents' generous pension, they were not eligible for the subsidy. The retirement homes I looked into were also different in that they ranged from independent to continued care. Some allowed for an independent lifestyle in which one would cook his or her own meals using a full kitchen in a condo- or apartment-style building. Others would be called Congregate Living accommodations in which the senior would have more companionship with the other residents by interacting with by sharing common areas and social activities, as well as dining together. However, they would also have a kitchenette for their personal use in their condo- or apartment-style facility. Assisted Living and Continued Care facilities allowed for a higher level of assistance to their residents. This ranged from things like bathing, dressing, laundry, meals and medications, and other daily tasks to twenty-four-hours-a-day assistance from nursing staff for those that have complex medical conditions and require routine check-ups.

I wanted my mother to be as happy and comfortable as she could be without forfeiting her much-loved independence or ignoring her declining health, so we settled on a compromise. We agreed to try and rent out her house so that she could still keep it, but I convinced her that her property would fall to shambles and her health would soon go with it if she wasn't going to welcome greater living assistance. The home that we chose was an apartment-like facility with a social room, exercise room, and elevators. This home had added security features to the building and premises but did not have staff available throughout the day. It was quite large so there were always daily activities in the common room.

The residents of each floor looked after one another by assigning a weekly monitor to make sure each morning each resident would hang something on their doorknob that said that they were inside the suite and were okay. If it happened that this token was not seen during the morning round, the monitor would call for help. Mom would still be able to cook her own meals at her full kitchen, which included an automatic timed shut-off. The bathroom was also nice that it had the appropriate devices to help both my mother and father with their mobility issues. This included many railings, a raised toilet seat, an extendable shower head and bathing stool, and an emergency alarm in case of accidents. It was great because all of this was in a decently sized abode of about 700 square feet. Not too big for my mother to clean and not too small for her to live in. This seemed like an ideal solution for the time being and I felt more comfortable that they would be able to spend time with other elderly residents.

They also had the option of regular meals prepared and served in a dining room downstairs, but my mother loves to cook and my father loves her cooking. She said that she will cook for him as long as she possibly can because Dad will not be pleased with eating something he's not familiar with. When I brought my parents to see the placed, my mother automatically fell in love with it and was already deciding where to put her things. We all agreed that this would be the closest thing to what they were comfortable with. The added benefit was that this facility was very close to where I lived, so I would be able to drop by and check in on how they were doing on a more regular basis, which they needed.

> *"This was the only way I knew to get my parents to leave a home they had lived in for over half their life. I know it must have been hard for them, like taking a part of their life away. But it had to be done, sooner or later. In this case, sooner is much easier than later."*

The day I sat down with my lawyer to discuss the power of attorney, he had mentioned that it would also be wise for my parents to think about what they want in their will. I really didn't want to think about what that implied, but I've heard horror stories about estate taxes and I wanted to protect my parents' finances. I brought them to a lawyer to help them update their will and let them allocate their assets as they saw fit. I found out that it was important to them that my children, their grandchildren, would have the ability to attend university. My mother started to get a little teary-eyed when she said this because she regretted not having been able to give me this gift after my graduation. Of course I told her not to worry so much about the past, and that I knew they did everything they could for me and more. I also mentioned that I had already started a Registered Education Savings Plan (RESP) for my kids and had been putting away what I could. But my parents would not hear it and wanted a portion of their wealth to go to both of their grandchildren. So they set up a trust fund, administered by their lawyer, to ensure they would be able to attend any university they wanted. This also allowed for the case that if my children did not wish to attend university, they would still be entitled to the entire portion of their inheritance to be put towards what they saw fit. This trust fund would then be unlike the RESP. In the case of an RESP, if my children chose not to go to a post-secondary institution, then the money that I contributed into the RESP would be returned to me. The remaining grants (contributions by the government) and interest (investment gains) go back to the government or are forwarded to a charity donation to a post-secondary institution. The drawback to the trust is that estate taxes will come into effect once my parents passed away. This means that the monetary gains within the trust will first be taxed by the government and then what remains will be given to my children. In this case as we thought it would be best to make their money work for my children. We had the funds placed into various investments. In essence, we didn't put all our eggs in one basket. I had to explain to my parents that this meant the children would receive the trust plus the investment gains less the percentage of estate tax. This estate tax on the investment gains cannot be greater than the income tax level of the deceased. For us this was the preferred method even with estate taxes taking effect.

After a few visits with the lawyer, she suggested that we also begin to look into the costs of burial and funeral expenses, which also gives us a good opportunity to talk about fulfilling the last wish of our loved ones. My mother was more concerned that we were not hit with one large expense at the end of her and my father's life. We decided to start putting away some of their pension to help with the costs. At the same time, we also began to look into the costs and which options my mother would want for the both of them. By this time my father had unfortunately degraded further and was in a too poor a state to be making any decisions. He was confined to a wheelchair for most of our outings and always had a distant look on his face. The three of us went to a funeral home in an attempt to gain a grasp on the many options available to my parents when the passed away. The first funeral director that we spoke with came on very strong and, to me, felt very much like a salesman. He wanted to convince us to purchase the best coffin and tombstone that was available saying that it really shows the impact a person makes in their life. When I politely refused, he made me feel like I was a selfish son by not wanting to give my parents the best in death. It wasn't until after the meeting, where I almost signed for a casket worth $5,000, that my mother had an extremely profound moment. She said to me "In the end the only thing that matters is that your father and I are together. You could put us in a wooden box and I wouldn't care. We have been together for so long… I want that time to continue in death." My mother's speech made me realize how poorly the funeral director had been treating me, making me feel guilty. We never went back

Capital Gains Investment
versus
Estate Taxation

Capital gains is money earned from purchasing different types of investment vehicles such as Bonds, Mutual Funds, Stocks, Options, or Futures. The money earned from GICs (as well as high-interest savings plans) is considered interest and taxed at your income tax level. However, in the former case, 50% of your capital gains is taxed at your income tax level. The third scenario is that Mutual Funds and Stocks may have dividends, another source of income from the purchase of these investments. The dividends you gain are taxed 20%.

Estate tax applies to the entire capital gain, or interest, or dividend of the investment. Estate tax on these earnings is taxed at the income tax of the deceased.

to that place and decided on a much nicer funeral director who did not pressure me to purchase the "Cadillac" set of caskets and to go with a more modest set.

I genuinely wanted to fulfill their last wish while they were coherent enough to make the decision, so we went to look at cemetery my mother had in mind. The final resting place for my parents was fantastic. It ended up facing the sun which the both of them loved. It was unexpected but my mother was the first of my parents to pass away, it came as such a shock since she had been in better shape than my father for so long but they found that she had passed away suddenly in her sleep. My father did not live for much longer before he joined my mother. When we moved him into an extended care facility he became unresponsive to the nurses and his health deteriorated at a brisker pace. It seemed that even in his late stages of Alzheimer's he still knew who my mother was and he was able to somehow connect with her. When her soul had left so had my father's. My mother was the one who was keeping him healthy and still mentally alive, despite everything. I cannot say that I didn't grieve when my parents passed. I loved them, envied them, and admired them. They were the quintessential couple. I know they lived a long, happy, and very fulfilled life together and even though it was difficult for them towards the end, they knew how important it was to me for them to make the decision for the people they leave behind.

––––––––––––––––––––––––––

☑   Canadian Pension Plan: This plan is not available to residents of Québec. To apply to the CPP you can either visit the Canadian Pension Plan website and apply or you can contact 1-800-277-9914. For residents of Quebec visit http://www.rrq.gouv.qc.ca/en/accueil/Pages/accueil.aspx

☑   Old Age Security: To get an application kit, you may contact them. For service in English: **1-800-277-9914** for service in French: **1-800-277-9915**, you may pick one up at a Service Canada Centre near you, or you can print one from the website

☑   Home Adaptations for Seniors' Independence (HASI): Contact the Canadian Mortgage and Housing Corporation **1-800-668-2642** and they will inform you on how to apply.

☑   Allowance Program: To apply for the Allowance Program you should call **18002779914**
TTY: **18002554786**

☑   Meals on Wheels: To apply for Meals on Wheels contact your local provider through your local yellow pages.

Resources

Federal/National Programs:

<u>Home Adaptations for Seniors' Independence (HASI)</u>

This program grants a refund of $3,500 for renovations to be completed on your home that improve access to the home and increase your safety. These renovations must be permanent fixtures to the home and the loan is applicable only if the work is completed by a licensed contractor. This program is provided by the Canadian Government and the Home Adaptations for Seniors' Independence, but you must apply through the Canadian Mortgage and Housing Corporation (CMHC). In order to qualify you must be 65 years of age or over and have difficulty with daily living activities due to loss of ability brought on by aging. Your total household income must be at or below the set income limit for your area and the renovation must be a place of your permanent residence. The application does not need to be completed by you, since it is possible for a family member to apply on your behalf. The full amount of the loan is forgiven to the homeowner if he or she continues to live in this home for at least 6 months; or forgiven to the landlord if the landlord does not increase the rent after renovations.

<u>**NOTE:**</u> This grant cannot be applied for after work has been completed, you need pre-authorization in writing from the CMHC before you begin to modify your home.

In the case of extensive modifications required to improve accessibility, such as wider doorways and increased space for wheelchair manoeuvring, the applicant for this program may also apply for financial assistance through the Residential Rehabilitation Assistance Program for Persons with Disabilities (RRAP-PD). Please see the previous chapters for more information about this program.

For information about HASI please see http://www.cmhc-schl. gc.ca/en/co/prfinas/prfinas_004.cfm

Additionally, you may also be eligible for assistance for a Secondary or Garden Suite if you are a low-income senior or adult with a disability. A secondary suite (also known as an in-law suite) is a self-contained unit with a separate entrance and full kitchen and bath within an existing home or added to a home. A garden suite (also known as a granny flat) is a self-contained unit that is not attached to the primary residence but built on the same property. The financial assistance for these types of domiciles is based on the geographic zone where the property is located, for instance, if you live in the Southern areas of Canada, the loan is $24,000.

For more detailed information about this program you can visit http://www.cmhc-schl.gc.ca/en/co/prfinas/prfinas_002.cfm

For information about CMHC programs and how to apply please call **1-800-668-2642**

Allowance/Allowance for the Survivor Program

This program, delivered by Service Canada, is a monthly benefit created for low-income seniors (aged 60 to 64) whose spouse or common-law partner is eligible or is currently receiving the Old Age Security (OAS) pension and the Guaranteed Income Supplement (GIS). You may also qualify for this program if your spouse or common-law partner is deceased and you have not remarried or entered a new common-law relationship for over 12 months. You must also have lived in Canada for at least 10 years after turning 18 and not be divorced or separated from your eligible partner for more than 3 months.

The table on the following page will help you identify how much you are eligible to receive and if you are over the income cut off point.

Caregiver Amount

This is a refundable tax credit for persons housing and providing in-home care for an elderly parent, grandparent, or other dependent relative of you or your spouse. You are eligible to claim a tax credit for each person you have within your home that you are looking after either alone or with your spouse. To be eligible the dependent relative must be at 18 years of age or older and have a mental or physical disability that is both severe and prolonged. In the case of parent or grandparent, the dependent must be born in 1945 or earlier. The dependent must also have a net income of less than $18,645. You are able to claim up to $1,062 of tax credits for each person you look after. This dependent must have lived with you for at least 365 days straight. You and another person may split this tax deduction but the total tax credit cannot exceed $,062. This amount can be claimed on Line 315 of your federal tax return. Additionally you will also have to complete and attach the appropriate part of Schedule 5 to this tax return.

For detailed guidelines and eligibility requirements, please see http://www.cra-arc.gc.ca/tx/ndvdls/tpcs/ncm-tx/rtrn/cmpltng/ddctns/lns300-350/315/menu-eng.html

You may also wish to contact the Canada Revenue Agency at **1-800-959-8281**

Allowance/Allowance for the Survivor Program Chart

Type of benefit	Average amount (March 2011)	Maximum amount	Income level cut-off	Income level cut-off for top-ups
Old Age Security pension	$495.68	$533.70	Not applicable	Not applicable
Guaranteed Income Supplement (GIS)				
Single	$458.58	$723.65	$16,176	$4,400
Spouse/common law partner of someone who:				
does not receive an OAS pension	$426.54	$723.65	$38,784	$8,800
receives an OAS pension	$288.36	$479.84	$21,360	$7,360
is an Allowance recipient	$375.90	$479.84	$38,784	$7,360
Allowance	$391.72	$1,013.54	$29,904	$7,360
Allowance for the Survivor	$588.18	$1,134.70	$21,768	$4,400

Provincial Programs:

Revenu Québec

This provincial organization provides information about income taxes, consumption taxes, tax credits, and provincial programs for individuals as well as deductions and contributions related to businesses, corporations, trusts, and organizations in the province of Québec. Outlined below are some programs of interest.

Tax Credit for Home-Support Services for Seniors

Crédit d'impôt pour maintien à domicile d'une personne âgée
This tax credit is to be used to help seniors retain their independence and reduce reliance on nursing homes for seniors. The program will pay 30% of the costs for home support up to $4,680, you may even use this tax credit to reduce your rental expense (max $500) or the amount you pay for condo fees. In order to be eligible for this program you must be over the age of 70 and be a resident of Québec.

For more information, please visit http://www.revenuQuébec. ca/en/citoyen/credits/credits/credit_remb/maintien_domicile/ default.aspx
You may also call Revenu Québec at **1-855-291-6467**

Shelter Allowance Program
Programme Allocation-logement

The shelter allowance program aims to provide financial assistance to low-income households who spend a disproportionate amount of their income on housing. It is eligible to individuals aged 55* or over, couples where one spouse is aged 55* or over, and families with at least one dependent child. The amount that is eligible will depend on the number of people living in the household, the type of household, income, and monthly rent. This allowance is calculated every year and paid monthly. You may be eligible to receive up to $80 per month if you qualify for the program.

*As of October 1, 2011, Revenu Québec will begin the process of lowering the eligibility age for this program, year by year. For the current year (as of October 1, 2011) the eligibility age will be 54 and reduced down to 50 by October 1, 2015.

For more information on this program you can visit the Société d'habitation du Québec webpage http://www.habitation.gouv.qc.ca/programmes/allocation_logement.html

Alternatively, you may visit the Revenu Québec webpage http://www.revenuQuébec.ca/en/citoyen/credits/programmes/programmes_Allocation-logement.aspx

You can also contact the Société d'habitation du Québec at **1-800-463-4315**

Régie de l'assurance maladie du Québec

This is Québec's mandatory insurance plan which includes Health Insurance and Health Care Services, Prescription Drug Insurance, and Financial Assistance. Below are some programs that are offered through this provincial plan.

Pension Plan Disability Benefits

To apply to the Québec disability pension plan go to the Québec pension plan website and fill out the application online. The criteria used to determine if you can apply for this pension is that you must have a severe and permanent disability (as recognized by the Régie's medical advisers), have contributed sufficiently to the Québec Pension Plan, and be under age 65. If you pass the criteria for a "severe and permanent disability" and if you are unable to perform a job because of your disability, then the pension would grant you at least $13,521 a year. However, if you are able to perform at a position that pays more than the maximum pension, which varies from individual to individual, you would not be able to receive this pension. The amount that a disabled person would be eligible for is $1,126.73 a month and the minimum that is paid out is $426.10 a month with additions depending on how much you paid into the Québec Pension plan.

Devices That Compensate for Physical Deficiencies

If you are covered by the Health Insurance Plan and meet the program's eligibility requirements, you are insured for the purchase, adjustment, replacement, repair and, in certain cases, adaptation of walking aids, standing aids, loco-motor assists and posture assists as well as their components, supplements and accessories; the purchase, adjustment, replacement and repair of orthotics and prosthetics. This program does not cover 3 or 4 wheel scooters, but does cover their repair.

Domestic Help Services

People using domestic help services provided by a domestic help organization that has been accredited for program purposes may be eligible to receive financial assistance towards the hourly rate charges.

There are two types of financial assistance:
- •basic financial assistance, $4 per hour of service, is granted to any eligible person, regardless of family income; or

- •variable financial assistance, $0.55 to $8.25 per hour of service, may be granted over and above the basic financial assistance, and is determined on the basis of family income and family situation

The maximum total assistance granted is $12.25 per hour of service ($4 basic and $8.25 variable). Any difference incurred between the rate charged and the amount of financial assistance granted is paid out-of-pocket.

Services that can be reimbursed are light housekeeping work, such as laundering, vacuuming, dusting, cleaning (refrigerator, bathtub, pantry, etc.); heavy housekeeping work, such a major cleaning jobs and clearing snow from the main access to the residence; preparing non-diet meals; and shopping for groceries and running other errands. There are some businesses who do not offer all of the services listed so it is best to find the organization that will be able to help you with what you need.

You are eligible for the program if you are over the age of 18 and if you are either a resident or a temporary resident of Québec within the meaning of the Health Insurance Act. If you are receiving any other financial assistance or compensation for these services under a different program you may only be eligible for a portion of the costs. To be eligible for variable financial assistance, you must be 65 years of age or over, or referred by a local community services center or health and social services if you are between the ages of 18 to 64.

For more information please see this website http://www.ramq.gouv.qc.ca/en/citoyens/contributionetaidefinancieres/exonerationaidedomestique.shtml

To apply, you may contact any accredited social economy businesses at the following website http://www.ramq.gouv.qc.ca/en/citoyens/contributionetaidefinancieres/eesad.shtml
You may also contact the Service de la contribution et de l'aide financières of the Régie de l'assurance maladie du Québec by telephone **1-888-594-5155** or TDD **1-866-820-8321**

Or by mail or in person:
Régie de l'assurance maladie du Québec
Service de la contribution et de l'aide financières
425, boulevard De Maisonneuve Ouest, bureau 213
Montréal (Québec) H3A 3G5

Coverage of Medical Services in Québec

The following medical services, including those that are rendered by a family physician or medical specialist, are dental services, optometric services, hearing devices, ostomy appliances, external breastforms, visual devices, and ocular protheses. For more detail about these services, please visit http://www.ramq.gouv.qc.ca/en/citoyens/assurancemaladie/serv_couv_queb/serv_couv_queb.shtml

Doctors who provide insured services

Most doctors participate in Québec's Health Insurance Plan, which means that insured persons who present their Health Insurance Card are not required to pay a fee. The Régie pays these doctors directly for the services they provide. You may wish to ask your doctor on whether he/she participates in the plan.

Some doctors have withdrawn from the Health Insurance Plan and do not accept the Health Insurance Card. Instead, they bill their patients for their services. In this case, patients must apply to the Régie for a reimbursement using a form obtained during the appointment and pay the fee upfront. These doctors are required to inform their patients of their status.

Other doctors, known as "non-participants", have opted out of the Health Insurance Plan and therefore do not accept the Health Insurance Card. The Régie issues no reimbursements for the cost of their services. They too must inform their patients of their status.

If you would like a list of health professionals who have withdrawn from or do not participate in the Health Insurance Plan, please visit The Régie's website at http://www.ramq.gouv.qc.ca/index_en.shtml

living on low income

Chapter 6

Chapter 6
Living on Low Income

When an individual is faced with a disability, he or she can simultaneously be faced with a physical burden, a psychological burden, and a financial burden. The financial burden is not unusual since there is not nearly enough government funding available. Often times, the burden is made worse by the accumulation of debt or a sudden change of circumstances in one's life or disability. Government funding acts as a safety net and may allow most disabled individuals to live reasonably well, but very meagrely. Government funding for disabled individuals and those with low income is by no means a source of income. Additionally, disabled persons, especially those that are new to their disability, are usually not able to work full time to support themselves let alone any dependents they may have. There may be no steady source of income and the insurance claim may not be substantial enough to live off of. To add to the ensuing financial problems, a vast majority of a disabled person's time is spent filling out paperwork so that he or she may continue to make financial claims to government sponsored programs and private insurance companies. The time that they spend could be put towards income-earning, but is forfeited to ensure their basic needs are met.

To address some of these problems, we have decided to give advice on how to overcome the hurdles them rather than criticize the situations. We have approached it with a series of questions and answers about living on low income and followed up with a guide on how to adjust to this lifestyle. This chapter is dedicated to those struggling to make ends meet for themselves, their families or others, whether you are disabled or not. We hope to teach you how to cope with low income and learn to live alongside it rather than becoming trapped in a cycle of debt.

Why

When faced with a life change, such as acquiring a disability which leads to a decrease of income, one must adjust their lifestyle to cope with the losses. Below are some of the necessities that one must pay for, but in turn can create a financial burden to most individuals:

What

1. medication
2. supplies (medical supplies or devices)
3. care services (doctors, specialists, home care nurses, occupational and physical therapists, chiropractors, masseuse, acupuncturists, psychiatrists)
4. housing (renovation versus renting)
5. decreased income (such as a job loss due to disability)
6. dependents, even if you, yourself, are a dependent
7. debt or no savings (even if your able-bodied partner may be able to make up the income difference)
8. re-training or re-educating for the work force in a job you're able to do

When

...can I start feeling comfortable about my financial situation?

The best way to feel comfortable is to set realistic goals towards achieving financial freedom. After a disability, you must re-evaluate the amount of income that will come into pocket, in respect to the amount of money that must leave. There will always be a time line of decreased spending up until you feel that you have reached comfortable living standards. Some people take years to adjust and some only months. Others may never achieve what they deem as a comfortable lifestyle but we hope that you may be able to find some security or balance and we hope that this guide will allow you to see at least some improvement in your financial situation.

How
...can I achieve financial stability?

The best investment a person can make is to consult a financial planner. A financial planner will be able to help you consolidate your debts and help you manage your savings so that you, your dependents, and your necessary expenses will be covered. If a financial planner is not an expense you can afford, government assistance programs may be available for those that live on a marginal income. It is also advisable that you try and implement some of the suggestions in the following guide to help you live on low income.

Where
...can I find help, resources, and info?

Many of the suggestions made in the guide below will contain internet websites or direct you in the right direction to get the additional information you are looking for. The guide is intended to be comprehensive enough so that you can grasp a basic understanding without going into unnecessary detail. Many topics are common-sense and others require a little bit of experimenting. If you required additional and more detailed explanations, most of the answers can be obtained via the internet or a financial professional.

Simple Tips to Saving Money:

1. Prepare home-made meals:

Food is a necessary expense that absolutely cannot be avoided. Unfortunately, it can also be one of the most expensive. Consider restaurant and take-out meals on a daily basis: on average, a decent sized meal for one adult can be $20 and up. One full day of dining out will set you back $60 minimum. One week of dining out is $420! That is close to the cost of one month's worth of groceries. Therefore, when possible, try to cook your own meals at home. There is a possible savings of $1260 per month just by enjoying some time eating in and preparing your own meals.

2. Before shopping, look for sales in local flyers:

Whether you are shopping for food or household items, the most important thing you can do before going on a shopping trip is to take a look online or through your local flyers for sales on the items that you might need now or in the near future. When possible, try to hold off on buying a material item that may go on sale in the future. If possible, substitute less expensive fruits or vegetables for the ones that might cost more. For example, if you had intended on buying apples, but saw that the nectarines were a better buy, then change your shopping list and buy the less expensive fruit alternative. Keep checking the flyers and sales and see if the apples are on sale next week. It is best if you able to go to a shopping complex where a variety of grocery, drug, and department stores exist so price comparing can be made. If it is not possible to shop at a large complex, don't forget to bring your flyer. Most stores will offer to "price match" a competitors price with a piece of proof, like a flyer. So, if Grocery Mart A has an item on sale that Grocery Mart B doesn't, go to Grocery Mart B with the flyer for the sale item and see if customer service will match their price.

3. Make a shopping list and stick to it:

The worst type of planning is when there is no planning at all. Before going shopping, make a shopping list on items that you absolutely need. When shopping, try not to deviate from this list, otherwise you may end up spending more than you had originally planned for. The only exception to this rule is finding a great sale on an item you will need in the future! But try not to make too many exceptions...

3a) SCOPs:

What are SCOPs? SCOP stands for Scanning Code of Practice. It is a general practice that many grocery stores nowadays are abiding to. What it gives the consumer is the item for free, if the item is under $10, or a certain dollar amount off if the price is above the $10 mark. This happens when said item's shelf label price is lower than when it's scanned in at the register. If you see that an item was marked on sale and it scanned in higher than tagged, let your cashier know, or take your receipt to the customer service and ask for a SCOP if your store follows this policy.

3b) Use coupons:

Coupons are everywhere and everyone should be taking advantage of them. Coupons are made for consumers like you and I to use—think of them as free money! There are coupons ranging from small values ($0.10) upwards to large values ($10, $20, $30 and up). There are the common coupons that are found at store shelves, or on products at stores, or given to you from the store on your next purchase, and there are coupons that are found in flyers and online, and online shopping discount codes. Coupons that are accepted must have a Canadian mailing address in the back. A coupon found at one store can be accepted at a different store, so it is not a bad idea to keep them for future use. However, beware of expiry dates. A store will not accept an expired coupon no matter what the excuse.

For more information about sales, coupons, and ways to save money try Smart Canucks http://www.smartcanucks.ca

4. Why pay full price?

Most of this section has been focused on not paying full price for any item you may be interested in. Now, I am going to suggest some alternatives to shopping at stores. Ebay is one of the biggest phenomenon of this century. You can find tons of items, new and used, at discounted prices. It is especially useful for certain electronics and designer items. Luxury items aside, Ebay is a great place to buy discounted clothes. One can find many brand new clothes for a very reasonable price, and usually the shipping costs are not too expensive because the parcel is light. The one thing to keep aware of is the cost of shipping. Always check the combined item price with shipping before bidding.

Another great place to find items is the classified section of the newspaper or on a classified online ad site. Kijiji is an online local ad service that is free for users to post items for sale or items wanted. Spending a little time to post a wanted ad, or browsing through some of these ads may save you quite a bit of money than if you were to purchase from store. Many items are also new or slightly used, and most people are able to negotiate on the price. There is also a barter or exchange section, where you may not need to pay in cash if you and the person selling are able to agree on items to be exchanged. During the summer, tons of yard sales and garage sales will spring up around your neighbourhood. If you have the time, check these out or make a list of close ones around your area. A trip around the neighbourhood can turn into a fun activity as well as a money-saving endeavour. Many of the items will be used, but I have heard of people getting many great lightly used items for free, or very close to free, especially at the end of the day. The best thing about this type of sale is that the sellers are usually willing to negotiate.

5. Free items:

Are you looking for something that you don't want to spend money on? One man's junk is another man's treasure. The Freecycle Network (http://www.freecycle.org) is a website where people in your area are getting rid of their unwanted items for pick up or delivery. Have you checked it out? A little rummaging through websites like these can turn up some items that you may be able to put to use.

6. Save on Gas:

Transportation is a considerably large expense for most people, especially when it is dependent for their livelihood. Public transportation is an environmentally- and financially-friendly way to save a few bucks, even if you only use it once in a while. Any car owner will tell you the hundreds they must spend to maintain their vehicle. Just to mention a few costly items include car insurance, maintenance (oil change, brakes, tire rotation or change), repairs, and gas. Need to get somewhere but don't always need public transportation? Try carpooling. www.carpool.ca is a great website full of environmentally-conscious people that are willing to offer a lift if you're heading in their direction! Many major cities also have a free service for pick-up and drop off transportation for people with disabilities or those with mobility problems. Call your local city official to find out of this program exists in your area.

7. Save on Electricity:

7a) Electronics:

Both small and large electronic devices drain power even when they are turned off. This is called phantom power and applies to electronics such as lamps, clocks, cable boxes, stereos, printers, fax machines, televisions, kitchen appliances, chargers, computers, and anything that is plugged into an outlet. To save on your electricity bill and to make your house more eco-friendly you can unplug the unnecessary devices from their outlets when you are not using them and when you leave the home for an extended amount of time, such a vacation. Also, be conscious of when you are not using a light in the house, a computer, or the television and switch off these devices. You will find that with a little persistence, overtime your energy bill will decrease and you'll feel a better about saving electricity.

7b) Air Conditioning:

During the summer months the cost of air conditioning can be a large chunk of the electricity bill. Those that have a basement are lucky to get away from the heat, but what if you are in a condo or apartment? Keep the windows open throughout the hot days, but keep the blinds or curtains closed. This prevents the sunshine from getting into your home where the heat will become trapped and accumulated. Keeping cold drink readily available in the refrigerator can also help cool you off. It's also important to keep hydrated when the temperatures are rising and you begin to sweat. If staying at home is not an option because it simply gets too hot, go out during the day when it is especially warm and hit the local mall, grocery store, or coffee shop. You can run errands or simply relax for a few hours, catch up with friends, and escape the heat.

7c) Heating:

Unfortunately, in Canada, we do require heating during the winter and this is a large part of the electricity bill during the winter months. Some ways you can save on heat during the winter is to have a timed temperature setting on your thermostat. For instance, you can have the thermostat set to turn off heat when you leave to go to work and turn back on one hour before you return. This method will save close to 8 hours of heating 5 days a week. Over a couple of years you could save a couple hundred of dollars by just applying this one method. Besides layering on tons of clothes and blankets when you're in the house, you can generate heat by doing a variety of daily tasks. Stove-top cooking and using the oven usually generate a sufficient amount of heat in the kitchen. The added benefit is that you can get your cooking done as well! Another simple way to generate more heat in the house is to use heavy curtains on the windows to trap in the heat that escapes from these fixtures. A simple and decorative way to keep your home or a certain room warm is to light candles. Even a few candles in a room can generate both heat and light which will efficiently limit your electricity use.

Save on Entertainment:

8a) Going for an outing doesn't always mean you have to spend a ton of money to have fun. There are plenty of summer and winter festivals or street fairs in each major city that are free to the public. If you are planning to stay indoors, why not host a pot-luck dinner party? Combining a pot-luck with any party is a great way to save time preparing appetizers and meals and save money on groceries! If weather permits, you can invite friends or family to a barbeque-picnic at a local park. Many city parks are free to the public but some require reservation. Plan ahead and you will be able to make your outing more enjoyable. Spend a movie night in by renting movies or borrowing from your local library. A library card is a good idea and an annual membership is affordable to most. You can borrow more than just movies from your local library. Television series, documentaries, music, books, newspapers, magazines and even the internet can be used or borrowed at your library. The library is a cost-effective as well as environmentally friendly way to reuse items that you do not necessarily need to have around the house. On the contrary, if you like the outdoors, try camping, or going for a hike, or simply an adventure outside at a national park where you can go canoeing, bird watching, swimming, or fishing.

8b) Are your children bored? Government sponsored programs such as the fitness tax for children. You may be able to claim up to $500 in tax credits for registering you or your spouse's child in a program prescribed for physical activity. This is a great way to get your children out of the house to make new friends and acquire new skills and experiences. It is also a great way to save a little even though you are spending. For more information about this tax credit, please see chapter 2 of this book. There are also lots of free youth groups and organizations that your children may be able to join. Other programs for low-income families are available for children to go to camps or be gifted with sports equipment that the family may not have otherwise been able to afford.

8c) If you are looking for affordable entertainment there are lots of web-coupon sites. How do these work? Companies that host these sites arrange with businesses to discount their products and services up to 90% of their original cost in exchange for advertising and the prospect of a large amount of purchasing from the customers. Many of these deal websites are specific to major cities and others may be online or international if they are offering a travel discount. Groupon (www.groupon. com) is one of the biggest and most commonly known deal sites out there. As an example on how this works, a local restaurant in your city may be offering $50 worth of food and drinks at a discounted rate of $25. This discount will be marketed on the deal website and is available to those with an account and credit card number. The account is free but all deal sites require a credit card to complete the order. The purchase is made and the website will either send you an email or update your account to print off your coupon to show the business or vendor when you claim your purchase. In this case, you will be able to order or purchase $50 worth of food, pay the difference if the cost is over this limit, and show the coupon to the restaurant to receive the discount. This is one of the best ways to enjoy your city and there are tons of different deals available every day. The types of deals are limitless, anything from professional services to travel. Just be aware that you verify the deal website and company is legitimate before giving out any personal information.

8d) Vacation:

If you are planning an inexpensive vacation you need to do some research before you go. Many flights and accommodations are dependent on the time you travel. High-season and low-season is dependent on the country of travel. Airline and hotel prices go up during high-season and decrease in low-season. If possible, try to plan your vacation during the low-season of your destination. By doing so, you can save a couple hundred dollars. Depending on where your destination is, the trip itself may not be as expensive as the food and accommodations. If you are looking for an inexpensive trip, try to find an all-inclusive vacation where your flight, accommodations, and meals are included in one flat payment. If you are travelling a short distance or if you do not have time restraints, you may opt to purchase a bus or train ticket. Weigh your options and see if this is a more affordable alternative to get to your destination.

9) Reward and Loyalty Programs:

A great way to save money or earn free items is to sign up for a reward program or a loyalty program. Reward programs are offered by a variety of different companies. You will find everything from food and grocery rewards to entertainment, travel, and household goods. Some of the bigger rewards programs in Canada are Air Miles and Aeroplan. The rewards obtained from these programs can be gift cards to a variety of stores, shops, and online merchants; travel mileage; household appliances; events and attractions; and other merchandise. Certain companies offer points for these programs if you purchase from them. For instance Safeway offers Air Miles on purchase and Sobeys offers Aeroplan miles. You may also be surprised that realty companies, car rental companies, and even travel companies will also offer Air Miles or other points if you choose to purchase their products or services. To date, there are 44 online companies offering Air Miles for purchasing from their company online. Other Canadian rewards programs include HBC/Club Z Rewards (The Bay and Zellers), PC Points (Loblaws, Superstore, Extra Foods), Esso Extra (Esso gas stations), Petro Points (Petro Canada gas stations), Shoppers Optimum (Shoppers Drug Mart), PetPerks (PetSmart), iRewards (Chapters, Indigo), and easyRewards (Staples Business Depot). Besides these companies, there are tons of companies that offer rewards for your loyalty to continue purchasing their product. Many loyalty programs offer a discount, a coupon, a gift card, or a free product after the purchase of a set amount of products from the same company. If you are unsure, it never hurts to check with a customer service representative to see if they offer rewards or loyalty programs

Some Tips on Making Money:

1) Hold a garage or yard sale:

Sometimes it is amazing to look through all of the stuff we've collected throughout the years. Its good idea to do a spring cleaning every year to figure out whether you will ever use all of the items that have piled up in the storage, the attic, or garage. What you will probably find is that a handful of items that are not or will not ever be used will go in the garbage, but you just might be able to salvage the rest and have a decently-sized yard or garage sale. This is great project especially if you are thinking of moving or renovating your house. It is really surprising how much you can make from the sale of items you would never think of using. A spin-off of this type of sale is a clothing consignment store. Usually, clothes don't sell well at a yard sale, but if you happen to chance on some gently worn items that were quite an expensive purchase you may be able to consign your clothing. If you were able to find only a couple of items and you think it is worth something (for example, a bike, home appliances, lightly used furniture) you can always try posting a free ad online at a website like Kijiji. Alternatively, you can also try posting an ad for bids on Ebay.

2) Online Surveys:

Believe it or not but some survey sites actually pay for your opinion! The payment is not a lot, but every little bit counts, and many people that do these survey actually enjoy doing them. They are usually not boring or tedious and are on a wide variety of subject areas. The only restriction is that some surveys are looking for particular groups of people, such as those that are in a certain age category or live in a certain geographic zone. Otherwise, most surveys are targeted to a large group of individuals. Companies that participate in this survey study could be anything from the Canadian government, a financial institution or a consumer product company. One of the sites that offers an honorarium for surveys is Survey Lion (www.surveylion.com). This site pays approximately $2 to $5 per survey and it selects applicants based on statistics that you given them. It is very simple to sign up and activate your account and you will receive invitations to surveys by email. Additionally you will paid for any referrals that you make for this survey site. This site will track your surveys after you complete them and pay you by mailing you a cheque.

3)Internet Surfing:

Do you spend a lot of time on the internet? Many websites are offering toolbars that allow you to gain points while searching the internet; the points can then be redeemed for gift cards or other items. This is a good way to earn free items that you may not have thought of purchasing, or gift cards that you may use on future purchases. Before signing up to use one of these services, you should always read internet reviews to see if the website is legitimate and reputable.

4) Mystery Shopping:

If you like shopping or dining and you have time and transportation, this is a great way to make some cash on the side. A mystery shopper is typically assigned to a location to evaluate staff on their customer service techniques. The establishment or company usually pays an out-sourcing company to hire mystery shoppers. Mystery shoppers are then sent out to experience and interact with the staff or personnel of the company they are evaluating and are then paid for their written evaluation. MS Job Board (http://www.msjobboard.com) is one of the mystery shopping out-source companies available. It is free to join and there are no requirements except your time and willingness to participate in a variety of environments.

Some Tips on Finances:

Chequing Accounts:

If you are on a budget crunch, try to open up a chequing account that does not require you to pay monthly fees or hold a minimum dollar amount in your account to waive those fees. Most of the large financial institutions such as TD Canada Trust, Bank of Montreal, CIBC, Royal Bank of Canada (RBC), and HSBC do not offer chequing accounts without a monthly fee. However, using a Student or Youth accounts may allow you get the monthly fees waived if these accounts are applicable to you. PC Financial is one such bank that offers free chequing accounts independent of income; they also offer free cheques. The disadvantage is that most of its services are done online or by phone and there are no active tellers to help you with transactions. PC Financial account-holders have access to CIBC's ATMs for free where you can perform most functions like deposits or withdrawals. They also have their own ATMs in Loblaws or Superstore grocery stores. By using PC Financial, you will also be able to earn points, something we will talk about a little bit later. Another option is to open a savings account instead. Some savings accounts do not charge fees, but the difference may be that you are allowed fewer transactions on your debit card or account for free. You will also not be able to purchase cheques under a savings account. If you cannot find a chequing account that is not free but is a necessity for convenience, try to look through your options and find one that allows you to maintain a minimum balance and hence, waive any fees. If you think that you cannot maintain a minimum dollar amount in your account, try finding a bank that offers very low monthly fees. If you are paying more than $5 a month, that is too much.

Tax Free Savings Account (TFSA):

If you have extra income available to you, you should try to take advantage of this type of savings account. The interest and investment gains earned in this account are not subject to taxation, however you may only put $5000 into this account per year. If you miss your $5000 contribution you can always add it in subsequent years. If you have never contributed, you currently have $15,000 in contribution room. TFSA's are the recommended way to save money. If you currently have a high-interest savings account, you should try to switch over to a TFSA. You may be able to get the same benefits and better, since your acquired interest will not be taxed. If you are debating between a Tax Free Savings Account and an RRSP contribution, figure out if you need access to the money in the immediate future. If you do, a TFSA may be the better choice since you are free to withdraw this amount most times without any penalty. If you are paying a significant amount of money on taxes, contributing into an RRSP may be more beneficial since it gives you a tax credit for the year. The best way to find out which money-saving strategy is best for you is to contact your local financial adviser. For more information about Tax Free Savings Accounts, please see chapter 7.

Registered Savings Plans (RSPs):

This will include the RDSP (Registered Disability Savings Plan), the RESP (Registered Education Savings Plan), the RRSP (Registered Retirement Savings Plan), and the SPRRSP (Spousal Registered Retirement Savings Plan). The benefit of putting money into the RDSP, as you may already know, is that the government will make its own contribution into the plan as long as you have the account open. The caveat to the RDSP is that you must be approved for the Disability Tax Credit before you may open an account. This type of account is primarily used to shelter your income and give you government grants. Similar to the RDSP, an RESP account will give you government grants while protecting your income as you save for your child's education. You may contribute to this account until your child or children reach 18 years of age. The downside is that if your children do not use the money in this account for post-secondary education, then the government grants will return to the government or go towards a post-secondary institution. The RRSP and SPRRSP are accounts that can help you reduce the amount of income tax paid to the government per year. The difference between the two is that your spouse cannot contribute to your RRSP and vice versa, however your spouse may contribute to a Spousal Registered Retirement Savings Plan (SPRRSP) on your behalf. You may continue to hold your own RRSP while contributing to your spouse's SPRRSP or while your spouse is contributing to your SPRRSP. The benefit of having a SPRRSP is if the income earned by one family member is significantly high and the RRSP contribution room in his or her account has reached the maximum. If this income earner wants to have an additional tax break, he or she may consider contributing to a SPRRSP where another tax credit will be issued to the contributor. The downside of these Registered Retirement Savings Plans is that the money cannot be withdrawn from the account, without being taxed, until the account holder turns 65. In the case of an SPRRSP you are the account holder if your spouse contributes into this account. The only other reason the funds can be withdrawn without taxation is if you are a first-time home buyer. For more information about Registered Savings Plans, please see chapter 7.

Pension Plans:

Pensions are a type of investment that accrue interest or investment gains while you hold this plan. The pension is to be used as another source of income upon retirement, however this income will be taxed when you use it. The Canadian Government has a pension plan called the Canadian Pension Plan (CPP). You will usually see this as a mandatory deduction off of your paycheque. Certain companies may also have private pension plans set up for their employees. Most often, these pension plans are voluntary; however, the benefit to contributing is that your employer may also contribute a certain amount to your private pension plan. Pensions are usually accessed when you declare retirement. The terms of retirement to private pensions will vary, so you must check with your company to see when these funds can be accessed. A good idea would also be to enquire about what happens to your work pension if you leave the company.

Debt Consolidation:

If you have credit card debt or loans you may consider debt consolidation. Debt consolidation requires you to take out a lower-interest loan to pay off your high-interest debts. For example, if you have debt on two credit cards, one with 18% interest and another with 20% interest as well as a student loan coming in at 5%, you may be interested in taking out a personal loan or line of credit (for example, at 8% interest) to pay off the credit card debt. However, you do not need to consolidate your student loan because the interest rate is lower than the personal loan. Over the long run, you will be able to save a lot more money to pay off your highest interest debt immediately. If you cannot acquire a personal loan, you may be able to use your mortgage as leverage. But in order to do so, you must own a property, whether it is paid off or not. To use your mortgage for debt consolidation, ask your mortgage broker if you can increase your mortgage. For example, if the amount of total debt on both of your 18% and 20% interest rate credit cards is $10,000 then you would ask to add another $10,000 on to your mortgage (that is at 4% interest). You can withdraw the $10,000 and pay off your credit card debt, thereby decreasing the interest you have to pay to only 4%.

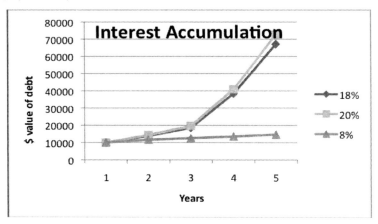

As you can see from the above graph it is wise to take out a personal loan at 8% to pay off even one credit card, since the interest that you save in the long run is significant.

Credit Cards and Debit Cards with Cash Back or Rewards:
If you are thinking about applying for a credit card you should consider getting a Cash Back or Rewards credit card. If you're going to spend money, you might as well get something out of it. You should be diligent and try to obtain one that doesn't require you to pay an annual fee, unless the benefit of the rewards or money back outweighs the fee. Rewards credit cards have a similar idea to rewards cards. For example, if you have a HBC Credit Card you can gain HBC points every time you make a purchase. These points can then be redeemed later for an item offered by the company. PC Financial has both a credit card and debit card that allows you to accumulate PC

points which can be redeemed towards a grocery purchase at a Superstore or Loblaws. Similarly, Bank of Montreal credit cards and debit cards allow you to accumulate Air Miles. Even gas companies have their own credit cards. Esso Extra allows you to accumulate points that can be redeemed at an Esso for gas, store purchases, or car washes. Some examples of Cash Back Credit Cards are the no annual fee CIBC Dividends Visa which gives you up to 1% cash back on eligible purchases. The MBNA Smart Cash Platinum Plus MasterCard gives you up to 3% cash back on eligible purchases with no annual fee. The "cash back" that you receive is dependent on the credit card company. They may pay this cash every year or every time you reach a certain dollar amount. They may pay it as a deduction on your credit card expenses or as a cheque mailed to your house. If you are thinking of getting a credit card that requires an annual fee, make sure you calculate how much you will spend per year versus how much you will be able to gain. For example, the Scotia Momentum Visa gives you up to 2% cash back on eligible purchases, however, the annual fee is $50. If you spend $2500 annually on this Visa you will be able to balance out the fee that you pay with the gain that you make. If you spend $3000 you will have a net gain of $10 (2% of $3000 is $60; $50 is spent on your annual fee). The easiest way to choose which type of credit card would benefit you is to take a look at your lifestyle. Do you travel a lot? If you do, paying for an American Express Gold credit card may be of more benefit to you than a Citibank Petro Points Mastercard. On the contrary, if you find yourself spending a lot of time driving, you may consider the Petro Points or Esso Extra credit cards. The most important thing to remember about every credit card, whether you have cash back or not, is to pay off the balance at the end of every month. With an 18% interest rate and 2% cash back credit card, you will not be able to gain back the amount you spend.

Payday Loans and Overdraft Protection:

The most important thing to remember about Payday Loans is to avoid them. The deduction off your paycheque can be as much as 15%, over the year it can be as much as 60% if you get a loan every two weeks. However, if you absolutely cannot wait until payday and need cash immediately, the best idea is to go to your bank and acquire a line of credit or overdraft. If you are running into financial problems more often than not you can consider overdraft protection from your bank. Overdraft is taking out more money than you have in your bank account and the amount that is allotted to you depends on your bank. For example, if you needed $800 immediately but your balance is $0 you may use overdraft protection to take out the $800, leaving you at -$800 in your bank account. This amount will go back to positive numbers when your paycheque comes in. TD Canada trust charges $3 per month for use of overdraft payments or $5 per use. An interest rate will be charged and will vary from individual to individual. If you find that you are in need of money every two weeks before payday, you should consider using the $3 per month option. If you find that you are in need of money every two months or longer, you can choose to pay $5 each time you need the money from your overdraft. A line of credit can be used for large amounts of money, however, you can choose to withdraw a small amount of money as well. If you apply for a line of credit you will be granted an allotted amount which you may take out a portion or a large sum or several portions. As mentioned before in debt consolidation, you may use this money however you want. The interest rate is variable and depends on each individual. A line of credit may cost more or may cost less than overdraft protection. For more information about these services consult your financial advisor or financial institution.

taxes
& the great
savings
vehicles of canada

Chapter 7

Chapter 7
Taxes and the Great Savings Vehicles of Canada

Now we will begin to talk about one of the two inevitabilities of life, which are death and taxes. Thankfully, with tax, you can avoid it. What we mean is that there are various ways in which you can lower how much you have to pay towards the government through legal tax avoidance methods. There is need to distinguish the terms avoid and evade. Tax evasion is illegal and there are severe punishments to those that are caught. Tax avoidance, however, describes methods on how to get around paying the full amount of your taxes. One act is smart and difficult to do; the other act is stupid and easy to do. Let us introduce the basic ideas of how you can be smart about government taxation without breaking the law.

The Tax Free Savings Account

The first step is to ensure that you are attempting to maximize your Registered Retirement Savings Plan (RRSP) contributions and your Tax Free Savings Account (TFSA) contributions ($5000 per year). The great thing about both of these savings vehicles

A TFSA is good for low-income families or the elderly. Any income or capital gains you achieve in the account are not considered taxable income. This means that you will be able to continue to claim either your pension or the NCBS at the same rate as before using the TFSA.

is that if you do not use your contribution room for the year, it carries over to the next year. The TFSA began in 2009, so first-time contributors are allowed the total of three years worth of contributions of $5000 each year. For example, if you do not currently have a TFSA, you will have the opportunity to deposit $15,000. If you decided you can only contribute $10,000 then the $5000 contribution room will carry over to the next year, giving you a total of $1000 ($5000 from previous year and $5000 from current year).

An excellent reason to have a TFSA is that if you make any monetary growth within the account, you cannot and will not be taxed on this growth. Although it is a small amount to start with, you have a chance to grow it every year. Even if you choose to invest in low risk Guaranteed Investment Certificates (GICs), which have guaranteed interest, you could see your personal wealth increase. Having said this, it is important to be aware of the amount of contribution room you have. The reason is that if you over-contribute, you will be taxed on this additional contribution until all of the additional contribution has been removed by tax or until more contribution room opens up.

Who is it for?

A Tax Free Savings Account is also an excellent resource if you have a disabled child who is over the age of 18. This account will allow your child to have a nest egg, should you pass away. On the contrary, if you are a disabled individual, then this is another way that you will be able to save. You might be wondering why would I choose to contribute to the TSFA when I can contribute to the RDSP? The answer is not that you should choose one over the other. The answer is that you should first contribute to your RDSP up until the point you max-out your contribution room. Thereafter, any additional contributions should be put towards your TSFA. The reason is that there is no benefit to contributing

> If you own your own company and work out of your home it is possible to claim a reasonable portion of your mortgage as a tax deduction.

more to your RDSP, especially since you cannot touch one penny in this account until a 10-year-period has passed. So therefore, the benefit to adding additional funds into the TSFA for your child or yourself is that you will be able to access the money in this account at any time, should any unforeseen circumstances occur. The downside of the TFSA is the limited amount of contribution room and the fact that there are no tax rebates or government grants should you choose to contribute into this account.

A TFSA is also a good idea for low-income families with dependent children and the elderly. Because interest or capital gains achieved in this account are not considered income, both these groups will be able to continue to claim government benefits without any deductions. For example, if a low-income family is investing within a TFSA and also receives money from the National Child Benefit Supplement (NCBS), the investment income that is gained within the TFSA will not affect the dollar amount of government support provided each month. However, if this low-income family is investing within a trading account and makes investment gains, the government will consider the money made as income and the dollar amount of government support from the NCBS will decrease. This is also true for those receiving pensions. If a senior invests within the TFSA and makes money, the government will not decrease his or her pension amount.

The Family of Registered Savings Plans

Another large savings vehicle that is offered to all Canadian citizens is the Registered Retirement Savings Plan or RRSP. The benefit to this savings vehicle is that any amount of cash you deposit into this account will give you a tax rebate. So long as you do not take any income from these accounts you do not run the risk of having to pay any taxes. The downside to this program is that, should you need to withdraw any amount of cash from this account, you will be taxed by the government and charged a fee by your financial institution. Withdrawing fro the RRSP is called "de-registering". Most investment firms keep a small percentage (10-30%) back of what you will owe (as taxes to the government), so always be wary when you have to "de-register" your funds. The purpose of the RRSP is to shelter any gains you achieve in the fund until you are 65 years of age (up to 71 years maximum). You are able to access your RRSP between the ages of 65 to 70 where this account will turn into a Registered Retirement Income Fund (RRIF). When you turn 71, the RRSP will automatically be transferred to a RRIF. A RRIF is an account which forces you to use the funds generated. You must take out a certain percentage of your RRIF every year and this amount will be taxed as income.

> The First Time Home Buyers Program allows you to withdraw $25,000 from your RRSP to be put towards the purchase of your first house. But be aware that the amount taken out must be re-paid in 15 years.

If you are concerned about how your child will pay for his or her post-secondary education you will be happy to know that there is another savings vehicle available with added government grants. You are able to save for your child's expenses at a post-secondary institution through the Registered Education Savings

Plan (RESP). This plan allows the contributor to put cash away, sheltering any monetary gains achieved within the account. The added benefit is that the account will receive government grants for the money is deposited. Like all registered savings plans there is a caveat to when you can withdraw the funds. In this case, you will not be allowed to take anything out of the RESP without proper documentation of your child attending post-secondary education. This plan enables you to save for the future much like the other plans. The bonus is that the account receives grants from the government which can be up to $7,200. This bonus is called the Canada Education Savings Grant (CESG) and the amount will dependent on family income. If your family is low-income, which means your family earns less than $72,000 annually, the RESP will receive an additional CESG on the first $500 of contributions each year. This additional amount is between 10 to 20 percent of the first $500.

There are additional education grants available to people living in Alberta and Québec. These two provincial grants are known as the Alberta Centennial Educational Savings (ACES or P-Grant) and the Québec Education Savings Initiative (QESI). All Alberta grants will require an application before you are eligible to receive any additional funds. To be able to receive the ACES grant your child must have been born or adopted on or after 2005. Under Alberta's program, an initial $500 is made to an RESP when your child is born, then additional payments of $100 are made when the child turns 8, 11, and 14 years of age. The Québec Education Savings Initiative (QESI) adds an additional 10% to your contributions up to a maximum of $500 per year.

For people that are disabled and currently receive the disability tax credit, the final savings vehicle began in late 2009. This, of course, is the Registered Disability Savings Plan (RDSP), a very special plan where the government will actually outpace your contributions if you are eligible. This is a great way to save and invest into the future as you are potentially gaining $3500 a year. Any gains that you make from your investments in this account are not taxable until you withdraw it.

It is important to note that you are not able to remove all of the government contributions at once. They must be taken out piece by piece after a certain time period elapses. The RDSP follows a 10-year-rule, so if you have received any government grant in the past 10 years, you are only allowed to take out the "minimum payment" which is described by a formula. The formula is the value of your account, divided by eighty, plus three, minus your age, plus all other payments you have withdrawn in the year. To make it easier to understand you could think of it as the value of your account divided by how long you are expected to live. For example, if your RDSP is worth $20,000 and you are currently 30 years of age and have not taken any RDSP payments out for the year, the maximum you would be allowed to take out is $377.58 [$20,000/(80+3-30)+0=$377.58].

The RDSP is meant to be a savings vehicle, but it can be set up to pay what is called an annuity. This is a set amount that is designed to last the length of your life. The best choice, if possible, is to wait until you have reached 60 years of age before you start withdrawing from the plan, since this method will give you the longest time to increase the value of your investments. As well, you should know that only the disabled beneficiary of the plan may withdraw funds. The funds cannot be taken by someone else unless the beneficiary passes away. In this case, the RDSP will go to the estate of the beneficiary. Once you have reached the age of 60 you must start withdrawing from the plan. There is a maximum limit to how much you are able to withdraw based on your life expectancy and how much your plan is worth. Also, you must file your taxes every year to continue to receive the RDSP grant offered by the government.

A really great website is **http://rdsp.com**. This site provides information on the RDSP, who qualifies and how to set one up, which financial institutions offer it, and an RDSP calculator that helps families realize the future value of having an RDSP. Additionally, much of the basic information to get you started is also available in French and Chinese. More detailed information including a step-by-step guide to registering for the RDSP is available through a free download on this site. The RDSP blog is updated frequently and there are telephone seminars available for guidance on this subject. While you are visiting this website, you should look into The Grey List, an excellent article which can be found by using their search bar. This article highlights the difficulties in applying for a disability tax credit and also what you can do to increase your chances.

Strategies for the Great Savings Vehicles of Canada

Compounding deals with interest, and how it can grow upon itself. It is the basis of many investment strategies and why the traditional "buy and hold" strategy is preferred. Let's use an example to illustrate this idea.

For instance, let's say that you will need to have $100,000 to look after your child when you have passed. This amount of money will allow your child to live in better care, but even if it was exceptionally managed, it would run out eventually. The principle of compounding is: The longer you have to save, the greater the impact of growth. We can compare this by looking at the option of having 20 years to achieve $100,000 versus 10 years. Let's say you gain 5% interest annually (which is a median monthly return when you investing in a broad selection of financial products such as mutual funds, stocks, bonds, and GICs). Over a 20-year period you would have to put away only $3024.26 at the start of year one to reach your $100,000 goal at the end of 20 years. If you only have 10 years you must deposit $7950.46 to reach $100,000. This amount is almost double the 20 year rate. To take it even one step further, if you only have 5 years to make $100,000 you would have to deposit $18097.48 which is 6 times the original deposit to get to the same amount. The main point that we want to stress to you, is that you receive the same benefit in the end. With proper planning you, not only have to save significantly less, there is also less stress for you to spend a greater amount of time to work for your money. You want your money to work for you rather than working for your money.

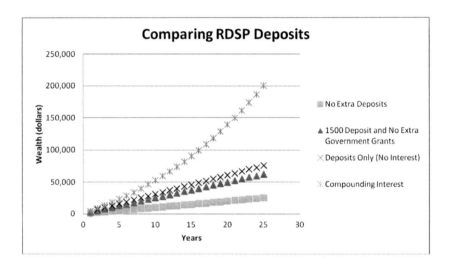

From the above example you can see the difference in the following graph between what compounding interest can do for you, as well as what depositing the maximum amount allowed each year can do for you.

Trading Accounts:
An Investment Rather than a Savings

A good investment vehicle to know is what is called a trading account. This account does not offer the same incentives as the accounts previously mentioned, but does offer tax breaks on monetary gains. Such gains can be made through dividends (a company's income paid to you) or through capital gains (you bought a stock that was worth $5 and sold it for $6). These accounts can also be "margin accounts", which means you can borrow money to purchase investments. However, there are downsides to utilizing margin since it is possible to be at a greater loss (in the negative numbers) than if you had invested using your own funds.

Trust Funds: A Sustained Benefit

Trusts are a valuable tool to ensure that an individual will remain eligible to receive government support even if they hold a large amount of assets. Some provincial programs require a disabled person to only have a small value in personal assets to receive ongoing benefits from the government. This is the case with British Columbia, which requires a disabled person to have fewer than $3000 in order to continue to receive financial support. In this case, it is wise to open a trust fund for this individual. A trust is a legal relationship between the creator of the account, the beneficiary, and a trust provider, usually a lawyer. The account is being held in trust to the beneficiary but does not belong to him or her. The only way the beneficiary can access the trust funds is to contact the trustee (the creator of the account). The lawyer for this trust fund will look for a financial institution or planner to manage investment decisions made on the trust fund. In B.C. an RDSP is considered an asset, so if an individual has $4000 in his or her RDSP, he or she will not be eligible for this province's disability aid. Therefore, it is a good strategy to circumvent the issue by opening a trust fund for your dependent. In addition to investments, the trust fund can hold property and other valuable assets.

What do I do with all these strategies?

Now that you have the tools to build the house, you need to know what type of materials to use! All of the above mentioned investment and savings vehicles are great places to shelter income to prevent it from being taxed. But what type of investments should you choose? Well, you have many, many options, each with their own risks and rewards. The first option you have is the least risky one and it is called government debt.

Government Debt that you can profit from

The first option you have has the lowest risk involved and that is government debt, which comes in the form of government bonds. Bonds mature at varying times; it will depend on the type you choose to purchase. When a bond matures, you are paid back the principle, which is typically $1000. In the case of government bonds, they are the only investment that will give you a guaranteed return and will not default (i.e. go bankrupt). However the downside is that the return (how much your money makes for you) is quite low, usually less than or only equal to inflation.

Banks need money too!

The next option that has a minimal amount of risk is called a Guaranteed Investment Certificate or GIC, this is offered by banks and other financial institutions as a way of getting funds from you, that they then loan out to other people. Base rate GICs typically pay at just about the rate of inflation or even lower, meaning that even though your money is gaining interest you are losing purchasing power (your money can buy less stuff because inflation is generally on the rise). For GICs you also have to wait for them to mature. The years to maturity will be stated when you purchase. It is also possible that a bank will go bankrupt. Not likely, but possible, that is why GICs have slightly more risk than government bonds. However, your investment is guaranteed up to $100,000, so if the bank goes under you do not lose your investment. There are other GICs that will try to match the return found on the common market, such as the TSX or other such stock markets. These returns can be higher than inflation. These GICs do not give you a guaranteed interest at maturity, but you will not lose any of your investment.

Can't choose one? You can have a ton.

The third type of investment is called a mutual fund. A mutual fund lets you invest in a group of stocks that are managed by professionals. Therefore, it indirectly gives someone else (the mutual fund managers) the control of your investment. What you have control over is the type of mutual fund you want and there are over thousands you can select from. You will also be able to see what types of stocks are in your mutual fund so you can get a better understanding of what you're investing in. A mutual fund is a great way to diversify your investments, thus limiting the amount of risk you are exposed to even if you are only using a small amount of your total investment. Diversifying limits risk because if one stock goes down and another goes up, you are thus, able to balance out gains and losses. Many banks offer mutual funds that cover various spectrums such as bonds and stocks. The great thing about mutual funds is that they take the worry out of choosing the "proper" investment and they allow you to be invested in different securities and gain a greater return versus investing in GICs or bonds alone. The downside is that you have to pay a percentage in management fees to the mutual fund managers.

You can take advantage of debt

The fourth type of investment is a bond; in essence, a bond is a company's debt. Bonds provide returns in two ways. The first way is that most bonds pay interest in the form of coupon payments, these are typically made every 6 months, but some pay every year or not at all. The ones that do not pay at all are called zero coupon bonds and you make money by holding the bond until it matures, which is when the company pays back its debt. The amount of a zero coupon bond that is paid out to you is more than you initially put into the bond. This is called capital appreciation and is one of the best forms of return due to the tax benefit where you are only taxed on 50% of the gains. The problem with bonds is that it is possible to lose the entirety of your investment if the company declares bankruptcy. This is why it is higher risk than mutual funds.

You can enrol your stocks in a program called Dividend Reinvestment Plan or DRIP which means whenever a dividend is paid from a stock you hold, and it pays enough to buy one whole stock of the same company you can receive the stock instead of the dividend. This is a great way to grow your portfolio no matter the condition of the market.

You don't need to be an entrepreneur to own a company

The fifth type of investment is called stocks. Stocks are a way that you can own a portion of a public company. Stocks are quite risky, even more so then bonds, as it is possible to lose everything you have invested into the stock because companies can go downhill really quickly. On the flip side it is possible to make a large return depending on your investment and the performance of the market, and thus the performance of the company. Stocks have the greatest upside but the most risk and we would only suggest investing in them if you can put in the time to find good companies. Always ensure you are not invested in just one stock, bond or mutual fund as you never know what will happen in the future. Good luck in your future investing and if you need help, always look for it from the professionals.

Tax Deductions:
Another way to save your hard-earned money

There are many disability-related tax deductions that should help you in your quest to remain independent and to build your own life. The first tax credit is the **Disability Supports Deduction,** which is only useable by the disabled individual. This may be used to deduct expenses that you incurred during the tax year that enabled you to go to work, school or perform any research that you received a grant for.

The Disability Amount (Disability Tax Credit) is another disability credit, however this credit may be transferred to someone else. It enables you to reduce your income tax if you qualify for it and includes a supplement if you are under the age of 18 at the end of the tax year.

The Disability Amount Transferred from a Dependant can be used when the disability amount cannot be claimed entirely by a dependent. For example, a child does not need to claim a tax credit so this amount can be transferred to the parent. Additionally, your spouse is disabled and is not earning or earning little income. You can transfer the full amount from your spouse or a portion, to use towards your tax return.

EMPCOLNULL

EMPTY

Medical expenses for self, spouse or common-law partner, and your dependent children born in 1993 or later: It is possible to claim medical expenses for yourself and your spouse/children on your tax return for various medical expenses incurred during the tax year. The expenses can range from an air conditioner to wheelchairs and wigs, however there are expenses that cannot be claimed such as cosmetic surgery, blood monitoring devices, gym memberships or health programs. It is also possible to claim "reasonable" moving expenses under your medical expenses if you are disabled.

It is possible that you do not have enough money, or insurance to purchase the medical devices that you require. If this is the case the best suggestion that we have is for you to look to the Red Cross who may be able to lend you the equipment you need at no cost to you. You do need to apply to the program through your local Red Cross, you are eligible if you are referred by medical staff and it is based on financial need.

You are also eligible to receive various tax credits depending on the province or territory in which you reside. This topic has been covered in previous chapters although not all provinces could be mentioned. The easiest way is to go to http://www.canadabenefits.gc.ca/ select the link that says "I am a person with a disability" and you will be able to select your province or territory of residence to find out more about programs offered.

Federal government supplements for disabled children

If you have a child who is disabled you may be able to receive government support in form of monthly payments. Obtaining Child Disability Benefit (CDB) is based on the Canada

Revenue Agency receiving confirmation from a medical doctor which states that your child has a severe and prolonged impairment in physical or mental functions. The CDB entitles you to a maximum of $204.58 per month for each disabled child. If you are making more than $40,726 net (after you pay taxes) then this amount will be reduced accordingly.

miscellaneous
information
to help you
make more informed
choices

_____

Chapter 8

Chapter 8
Miscellaneous Information to Help You Make More Informed Choices

Employment Insurance

Employment insurance (EI) is a valuable tool that enables you to receive income if you have lost your job. It is based on your previous full year of employment (1 year from the termination date of employment) so as long as you have worked for at least a year you are entitled to receive EI. It is very easy to apply and create your EI account either through the internet at http://www.servicecanada.gc.ca/eng/ei/menu/eihome.shtml or in person at any service Canada location in your city. The online application is very easy to fill out and there are only a few things you will need. The most important information you will need that you may not have is your record of employment. The record of employment can be requested from your previous employer and they have to provide it to you or send it to Service Canada (usually your company's human resources department will know where to send it). The second document you will need is your social insurance number; then you can begin the application. It is a very straight forward questionnaire, and if you have any questions you can call Service Canada at **1-800-206-7218** (TTY: **1-800-529-3742**).

Even if you were terminated from your previous position you usually will be eligible for EI. The number of weeks that you can receive EI and the amount you can claim will depend on the area that you live in and your income for the previous year. The maximum time you can claim EI is 52 weeks, although it can be shorter if your area has low unemployment. There is an EI claim waiting period of 30 days from the day of employment termination. The faster you start your application the faster it can be completed. It is also beneficial to apply as soon as possible because after a certain period of time, you will no longer be able to claim EI. After the 30 day waiting period is over EI pays you in arrears or in other words pays for the amount of time that you have not worked, so for those full 30 days you will be paid depending what your record of employment shows and whether or not you have been able to find employment again. It is also important to note that your employer is required, by law, to provide you with your record of your employment.

Once you have applied to EI you have to submit regular reports indicating if you have found work and if you have made any income. Income from stocks, bonds and mutual funds do not count to this amount so it is possible to receive both EI and income from selling stocks, although you must be careful to inform the government if you are going to be a full-time day trader and that would take you off of EI. These reports are due every 2 weeks and are very straightforward, with only 6 or so yes or no questions that can either be filled out online at the Service Canada website or you can call the number listed above. Sometimes you will be required to contact Service Canada, depending on your answers to the questions.

If you ever lose your job it is important to begin applying to a new position within your field as soon as possible. Although, we suggest that if you were let go, to take a couple days and relax before you begin the task of job applications. There are numerous websites that will aid you in your job search such as Workopolis (http://www.workopolis.ca), Monster (http://www.monster.ca) and many others around the web. The trick to job hunting is not to be discouraged, you will send out many applications and get many rejections you just have to keep working at it. Another resource to use is Temp Agencies, they provide temporary work to allow you to continue in various jobs and prevent you from having a large gap in your resume where you have been unemployed.

For the disabled, there are other options as well, throughout this book you have seen various programs that will help you become prepared for employment and even help with training and finding a job. Use all of the resources that you have at your disposal and it will greatly increase your chance of gaining employment in a field you want.

<u>The Interview</u>

One of the trickier parts of the job hunt is actually doing well in the interview. I would suggest that if you get the chance to be interviewed, even if it is for a position you have no desire to take, still take this opportunity as a chance to the practice your interview skills. You will better understand what type of questions you may be required to answer. As well there is never any harm in trying to glean information from the interviewer by having some questions prepared for the interview before hand. Make sure you do some research on the company you are being interviewed by, since it seems they always like to know what you have heard about their company. Research and prepare against the basic questions that you hear in almost every interview such as "What are your skills?" and "What are your weaknesses?" For weaknesses there are different schools of thought on what you should say, some people believe it is best to give a weakness that is really a strength such as being a perfectionist and therefore taking your time with your work. Other people believe it is best to give a weakness and then give details on what you are doing to improve or fix that weakness. It is up to you on what you feel will serve you best in your interviews, and what you sense from your interviewer.

Self-Employment: Make it Work for You

If you do not want to work for someone else you can always work for yourself and disabled individuals gain access to the government program **Entrepreneurs with Disabilities.** This program is strictly for western provinces and is delivered through the Community Futures organization. This program offers mentoring and one-on-one counselling services, access to business training and development, help to identify requirements for specialized equipment, and business loans. In order to be eligible for assistance you:

1) Must prove that you have received funds from other sources such as banks or capital venture firms in the past
2) Are restricted in your ability to perform at least one of the basic activities of entrepreneurship or self-employment
3) Are disabled due to physical or mental impairment and
4) Have a viable business plan and are a new or current small business owner with a disability.

The loans that are provided are flexible and help you if you cannot receive loans from traditional sources such as banks or other financial institutions. If you would like to know more, contact the Communities Futures at:
http://www.communityfuturescanada.ca/

Fraud and How to Avoid It

Fraud is an area that has been receiving a greater portion of our attention due to the various methods that nefarious and cruel people attempt to dupe individuals out of their hard earned income through deceit and lies. Fraud not only affects individuals but companies as well. There are various ways to protect yourself from fraud. If something sounds too good to be true, then it is not to be trusted, or at the very least, look deeper into what the

One of the reasons for the increased difficulty of receiving the Disability Tax Credit has been due to fraudulent applications for the tax credit from organizations who apply on a person's behalf, charging a small fee.

program offers and evaluate peer reviews. For instance, a quick Google search will often lead you to various web sites slamming the apparent scam and the method on which they deceive people. Some other ways to protect yourself is to protect your personal information: Social Insurance Number, Driver's Licence, Credit Card Numbers, Phone Number and sometimes even E-mail Address. by being smart about who you give the information to, as well by protecting your credit card and debit card PIN whenever you purchase anything. For instance many financial companies will ask for your information when you initially set up a account in order to verify your identity, but will not contact you specifically to ask you over the phone for these details.

Fraudsters have been increasing their use of the internet to gather your personal information. For instance, if you receive an E-mail from your bank indicating that they believe your account has been compromised and they wish for you to sign into your bank account online, this is highly suspicious. This is what is called a "phishing" scam and the link the E-mail provides you with will go to a website to capture your personal information. It will look exactly like your bank's website but when you enter your information, the site will give you errors. Most likely, you have just given criminals access to your bank account. If you are ever in doubt whether your bank account has or has not been compromised, call your bank. The number to use will most likely be on the back of your credit or debit card. If you are receiving a phone call from someone that claims to be your bank, but the person is asking you personal information, do not respond, even if they say they are trying to find out if your account has been compromised. The best thing to do is hang up and call your bank at the trusted phone number they have given you. Credit card and debit card companies, under normal circumstances, will not contact the account holder and ask for personal information.

Another scenario that has targeted the elderly is a phone call from a distant relative that states he or she is in trouble and needs money. This phone call will often sound very personal and the person on the other line may sound like they have intimate knowledge of your life, calling you "Mom" or "Grandpa" or any other familiar names. They can even pretend to be your lawyer or another trusted professional as it is very easy to obtain a person's name, simply by going through their mail or the phone book. Again, do not, under any circumstances, give out personal information. Refrain from doing so even if this person says he is your grandson, he has gotten in trouble with the law, he is across the country, and needs a wire-transfer to post bail. Fraud comes in infinite scenarios and takes many forms, so always yield on the side of caution.

———————————————

We hope that this book has provided you with many tools that have enabled you to succeed in your life and gain greater personal and financial independence. We also hope that with all the information contained here you have been able to learn that there are many different programs available to you and different methods to help you through your disability, whether great or small.

About the authors:

DR. AUSTIN MARDON was born in Edmonton, the son of Ernest and May Mardon. Educated at Lethbridge University, he did a M.A. at South Dakota State University and his Ph.D. at Greenwich University, Australia. Dr. Mardon also served as a research scientist and participated in a meteorite recovery expedition with NASA in the Antarctic. Since then, he has been involved with humanitarian efforts and advocating for those with mental illness. His work to help those who suffer from schizophrenia has helped him earn an appointment to the Order of Canada in 2007.

SHELLEY QIAN and **KAYLE PAUSTIAN** were raised in Edmonton and are currently working and residing in Calgary, Alberta.

Shelley is a pharmacology major from the University of Alberta who aspires to become a veterinarian. Her interests range from the medical field to the financial and she enjoys volunteering her time for a variety of causes.

Kayle holds a bachelor of commerce degree from the University of Alberta. He is working towards completing both C.F.A. and C.M.A. designations. When he is not studying, he enjoys reading, investing, and outdoor activities.

About the editor:

LAWRENCE DOMMER was born in Grande Prairie, Alberta, before moving to Edmonton to attend the University of Alberta, where he earned a Bachelor of Music and a Bachelor of Education. Currently, he resides in Grande Prairie and works as an educator while volunteering in his spare time.